CW01522044

AIDS and
SYPHILIS
The Hidden Link

AIDS and SYPHILIS

The Hidden Link

by

Harris L. Coulter, Ph.D.

North Atlantic Books
Berkeley, California

Wehawken Book Company
Washington, D.C.

AIDS and Syphilis — The Hidden Link
by Harris L. Coulter, Ph.D.

Copyright © 1987 by the Center for Empirical Medicine

ISBN 1-55643-021-3 (paperback)
ISBN 1-55643-025-6 (cloth)

Published by:
North Atlantic Books
2320 Blake Street
Berkeley, California 94704
and
Wehawken Book Company
4221 45th Street N.W.
Washington, D.C. 20016

Cover and book design by Paula Morrison
Typeset by Classic Typography
Second Printing, 1987

AIDS and Syphilis — The Hidden Link is sponsored by the Society for the Study of Native Arts and Sciences, a non-profit educational corporation whose goals are to develop an ecological and crosscultural perspective linking various scientific, social, and artistic fields; to nurture a holistic view of arts, sciences, humanities, and healing; and to publish and distribute literature on the relationship of mind, body, and nature.

Library of Congress Cataloging-in-Publication Data

Coulter, Harris L.
    AIDS and syphilis.

    1. AIDS (Disease)—Etiology.   2. AIDS (Disease)—
Immunological aspects.   3. Syphilis—Chemotherapy—Com-
plications and sequelae.   I. Title.
RC607.A26C68   1987   616.97′92071   87-21961
ISBN 1-55643-025-6
ISBN 1-55643-021-3 (pbk.)

Contents

And this disease of which I speak, this syphilis too, will pass away and die out, but later it will be born again and be seen again by our descendants just as in bygone ages we must believe it was observed by our ancestors.

Girolamo Fracastoro (1484–1553)

Introduction

AIDS was first identified in 1981 in Los Angeles.[1] The UCLA Medical Center reported five young homosexual men suffering from a pneumonia of unusual origin; the causal microorganism — a protozoon known as *Pneumocystis carinii* — was regarded as ordinarily innocuous and, in fact, is found in nearly all healthy persons but for unfathomable reasons had suddenly become lethal. Such an outcome had previously been noted only in persons undergoing immunosuppressant therapy, whose immune systems had been undermined by cancer, or who were severely malnourished.* Soon it became clear that these peculiarly severe cases of pneumonia were occurring in individuals with shattered immune systems.

This same pneumonia turned up in New York as well, together with several dozen cases of an unusual skin cancer called Kaposi's Sarcoma which had previously been almost unknown in the United States.

Eventually *Pneumocystis carinii* pneumonia (PCP) and Kaposi's Sarcoma (KS) were interpreted as secondary manifestations of an underlying immune-system deficiency of unknown origin which was called "acquired immunodeficiency

---

*"Immunosuppressant therapy" means the use of drugs which suppress the body's inherent tendency to fight against any substance which it recognizes as not part of itself. Immunosuppressant therapy is commonly used after skin and organ transplants, to prevent "rejection."

syndrome" or "AIDS."

The first few thousand cases were found overwhelmingly in homosexuals, and AIDS was initially called "Gay-related immune deficiency" (GRID), the "Gay plague," etc. But in 1983 it was found to affect heterosexuals as well.[2]

To date more than 37,000 cases have been reported in the United States, with over 21,000 deaths.[3] The cumulative mortality is 58% after six years. The Public Health Service has estimated that in this country up to 1.5 million persons may carry the virus alleged to be the causal agent; Surgeon General C. Everett Koop states that the actual number is probably "much higher." The figure worldwide is estimated in the tens and even hundreds of millions.[4]

The groups who feel particularly threatened are panicked at the thought that the epidemic will just grow and grow. The Public Health Service warns that by 1991 the total number of cases worldwide will reach 300,000, and of deaths — 179,000; over 50,000 deaths are predicted for the United States — and will bring AIDS level with automobile accidents as a leading cause of mortality. Furthermore, the treatment of these patients will cost from $8 to $16 billion per year.[5] An official of the Department of Health and Human Services voiced the general feeling of nervous edginess in calling these figures "staggering" and "devastating."[6]

In Africa, where AIDS is already epidemic, if the present morbidity and mortality rates continue, the catastrophe will be even more terrible, and by the end of the century substantial portions of the population will die in Zaire, Rwanda, Uganda, and their neighbors.* Dr. Halfdan Mahler, head

---

*"Morbidity" means the tendency to fall ill. The "morbidity rate" over a given period of time, such as one year, means the percentage or proportion of the population which will fall ill during that year. The "mortality rate" means the percentage or proportion which will die during that period.

of the World Health Organization, has called AIDS "a health disaster of pandemic proportions" and said he could "not imagine a worse health problem in this century."[7] A Harvard biology professor has raised the ante still further, warning that the disease might ultimately carry off "a quarter or more" of the world's population; thus the promised devastation is supposed to equal that of the Black Death in the fourteenth century, which killed a quarter of the human race.[8]

As we will show, these prognostications are undoubtedly too pessimistic, but, even if a quarter of the earth's population does not perish of AIDS, there will probably be millions of deaths.

This has been an unexpected shock to both physicians and the public. No respectable scientist in 1980 could have imagined that an incurable epidemic was about to be visited on mankind. Hence their reaction has been unsatisfactory. When confronted with a terrifying challenge, individuals and social groups revert to primitive responses. Unable to realize that AIDS is a qualitatively different phenomenon, physicians and scientists have equated it with other conditions medicine has conquered in the past — caused by a virus or other microorganism and yielding to the appropriate "magic bullet" in the form of a drug — or perhaps a vaccine.

If everyone infected with the AIDS virus is doomed sooner or later to contract the disease and die of it, the prospects are apocalyptic. Existing efforts at countering the epidemic seem to assume this. The prevailing view is that in time nearly all who are infected with the virus will come down with the disease.

In the following pages we take exception to this view. We doubt that a substantial portion of those with the virus will ever become sick with AIDS. We also dispute the possibility of curing AIDS with a drug or vaccine directed against the supposed viral cause. Instead we outline a new interpretation of the genesis of this cataclysmic disease and indicate ways of coping with it, of limiting and averting its further depredations. In particular, we indicate guidelines for preventing the emergence of new cases.

Instead of the analytical and reductionist approach to this problem which is favored by the medical establishment, we propose a historical and synthesizing one. Instead of seeking to pinpoint a viral "cause," we examine the factors enabling this "cause" to act. It has probably always been present in some population groups, who have learned to live peacably with it. The question is why, in other groups, it suddenly became lethal.

Even if, as we believe, the AIDS epidemic will eventually level off, much can be done to assist the process. But this will demand new thinking about some fundamental issues in medicine. In particular, physicians will have to scrutinize their therapeutic procedures and ask searching questions about techniques in use since the dawn of the antibiotic age in 1945.

The threat of AIDS should stimulate new medical thinking. The epidemic should be seen as an opportunity to re-evaluate some of the medical truisms of past decades.

1

Microbe
or Host Organism?

The history of bacteriology has seen an ongoing clash between scientists who stress the overriding significance of the bacterium, virus, or microbe as the disease "cause" and others who emphasize that no microbe infects everyone exposed to it. The first group, headed initially by Louis Pasteur, has sought to cure disease by identifying this "causal" microorganism and destroying it. The second group, led by Pasteur's opponent Antoine Bechamp, resolved that the condition of the "host organism" determines who falls ill and who does not. They advocated treating disease by strengthening the resistance of the patient.

The emergence of any new disease on the medical scene inevitably resuscitates this controversy.

Since AIDS was seen as a discrete and different disease, medicine's instinctive reaction was to seek a new cause. Because it appeared to be infectious and transmissible by blood transfusion, the search soon turned to a virus which could be passed on in this way. In due course this led to the discovery (simultaneously by Robert Gallo in the United States and Luc Montagnier in France) of a microorganism called variously "human T-cell leukemia/lymphoma virus," "lympha-denopathy-associated virus" (LAV), "human T-lymphotropic virus type III" (HTLV-III), "AIDS-associated retrovirus" (ARV), and, most recently, "human immuno-deficiency virus" (HIV) or simply, "AIDS virus."

By whatever name, it is thought to invade the tissue of the immune system and cause its collapse, leaving the body helpless before infections which otherwise it could easily repress.[1]

Antibodies to this virus — signs of the body's reaction to previous infection taking the form of bits of protein in the bloodstream — have been found in many AIDS patients, and this seemed to settle the question of causality.[2] A recent publication on AIDS coauthored by Gallo and other authorities concentrated attention entirely on the virus.[3]

But this is an old-fashioned way of thinking. If the virus had not existed, it would have had to be invented.

In fact, the theory of a single AIDS-causing virus started eroding almost as soon as it appeared. In November, 1986, Montagnier announced discovery of a new AIDS virus, which he baptized LAV-2 or HIV-2, claiming that it was the major cause of AIDS in the countries of West Africa. Later that same month yet another AIDS virus was discovered in West African AIDS patients being treated in Sweden and was provisionally called SBL 6669 V-2 in honor of the Swedish State Bacteriology Laboratory.[4]

These discoveries have necessarily detracted from the "one microbe, one disease" assumption originally at the root of AIDS research. Montagnier alluded to this in his announcement: "This finding was really a surprise to us. I couldn't imagine two viruses causing the same disease."

Gallo and Montagnier have admitted that more AIDS viruses may eventually be found. But if AIDS turns out to be associated with a dozen or more viruses, this necessarily detracts even more from their significance as causal factors and shifts attention back to the host organism.

Indeed, under laboratory conditions the original AIDS virus seems not even to possess a high degree of toxicity. In 1984 scientists at the National Institutes of Health (NIH) and the Centers for Disease Control (CDC) injected chimpanzees with samples of blood from AIDS victims or with pure cultures of the virus itself. None of the monkeys died, some were apparently unaffected, while others developed mild symptoms resembling those of AIDS-related infections.[5]

There have been hundreds of reports of healthy physicians, nurses, and hospital workers accidentally sticking themselves with virus-infected hypodermic needles and suffering no consequences at all. At the most they have come down with a condition resembling infectious mononucleosis which resolves after a couple of weeks. None has died from AIDS or even become sick with it.

Such experiments and accidents hardly justify calling this microbe a "killer virus." Furthermore, it cannot even be isolated from about half of the patients, while antibodies to it (indicating previous or ongoing infection) are not found in 10 percent.[6] The virus cannot be detected at all in cases of Kaposi's Sarcoma.[7]

AIDS must be seen as a dynamic interplay between infection by the causal microorganism and the resistance of the host. In the healthy individual few germs can get a foothold. As host resistance declines, increasing numbers of once friendly, or moderately hostile, microorganisms become virulent, and the severely weakened patient can die of a common cold.

The AIDS virus is probably little more than another "opportunistic" infection of an *already destroyed* immune system — at the most a "co-factor" which may possibly give rise to AIDS when combined with other factors.

This is already known to be true for PCP. The *Pneumocystis carinii* is found in more than 95 percent of healthy persons and is life-threatening only in the individual with a defective immune system.

According to the accepted wisdom, this happens when

3

the immune system is first destroyed by the AIDS virus. But what is true for the PCP microorganism may be equally so for the AIDS virus. Perhaps *both* can get a foothold only when the immune system has already been compromised. If so, the search should be for factors which undermine the immune system and thus predispose to infection with PCP, the AIDS virus, and others which may ordinarily be quite innocuous.

The following pages discuss a disease — syphilis — which can readily cause immune collapse and thus usher in a case of AIDS, but whose role in the current epidemic has been almost totally ignored.

2

The Syphilis Connection

Syphilis, a disease caused by the *Treponema pallidum*, erupted in Europe during the waning years of the sixteenth century. Because the outbreak coincided with the return of the Columbus expedition from the New World, his sailors were blamed for picking it up from the Caribbean Indians, but no one really knows if that is true. The plague was phenomenally virulent in the initial decades, with many dying within weeks or months from its acute effects.

In following centuries it passed into a chronic form and became an ever-present fact of medical life everywhere in the world, no longer fearsome for its immediate lethality but still dreaded for its capacity to cause long-term disabilities. A study of untreated syphilis in Norway in the early 20th century found that 70 percent of the patients recovered entirely without any treatment at all, 15 percent suffered chronic incurable cardiologic and neurologic damage, and another 15 percent had symptoms which were relatively benign. There was a slight excess mortality, as compared to healthy persons, but, on the whole, these syphilitics lived to a ripe old age.[1]

During the First World War medical commissions in both

England and the United States estimated that between 10 and 20 percent of recruits showed signs of infection; this probably represented the extent of syphilis infection in Western societies at that time, although some authorities thought it was marginally more prevalent in the United States than in Europe.[2] As late as 1986 a survey in England of almost 2000 hospital patients over 55 years of age found that 2.5 percent showed signs of previous infection with syphilis; three fourths of them had never been diagnosed or treated.[3]

In 1945, when the new medicine, penicillin, seemed to promise a total cure, it was allocated to treating this ancient scourge. A massive campaign was unleashed in the United States; a network of Rapid Treatment Centers was set up, and millions of dollars of federal funds were appropriated every year for purchasing this still scarce and expensive drug.[4]

Initially, the campaign seemed successful. Between 1948 and 1953 the number of new cases declined from 106,000 per year to fewer than 10,000.[5] When treated in an early stage the patient felt better, his symptoms disappeared, and he seemed cured. But, because the benefits of penicillin appeared so obvious, no controlled study was ever done to determine if the new drug was truly curative; "clinical impression" remained the basis of the positive evaluation of penicillin treatment. In particular, no large-scale or sustained effort was made to investigate the long-term consequences of treatment—to ascertain how healthy these "cured" cases really were.[6]

This was a mistake. In the early 1960's, to everyone's surprise, new cases started to increase, and it became evident that the relationship between syphilis and penicillin is less straightforward than physicians had assumed in the first promising post-war years.[7] Syphilis incidence in the United States peaked at 25,000 cases in 1965 and just over 32,000 cases in the early 1980's; it has declined slightly since then.

The reasons for the increase have been much discussed, and the consensus is that (1) the apparent elimination of syphilis as a health threat contributed to sexual liberalization, whereas (2) syphilis was not really eliminated at all, merely disguised and masked. It remained a source of infection which was revitalized by the relaxed sexual attitudes of the 1960's and 1970's.

□ □ □ □ □

What is more, syphilis prepared the ground for the emergence of AIDS.

From the very beginning the typical AIDS patient was likely to show evidence of previous infection with this disease.

Here homosexuality is a good place to start. About three quarters of AIDS victims are individuals following the "gay lifestyle." But this lifestyle is very often associated with syphilis, especially in the male. In the United States today the homosexual male is 14 times more likely to have had syphilis than the heterosexual male; 75 percent of syphilis cases are in males, of whom almost half are either bisexual or homosexual.[8] Thus, a CDC spokesman could state in 1985, "Gay men account for more than half of the syphilis in the country."[9]

Two extended studies of homosexual AIDS patients with KS or PCP reported to the CDC found a high incidence of previous syphilis infection. A 1983 survey of 50 cases, with the patients being questioned closely about their medical history, found that 68 percent showed signs of previous syphilis; it was the second most important risk factor for acquiring AIDS after "number of male sex partners per year."[10] In 1984 this group was compared with 31 heterosexual AIDS patients, this time using laboratory tests for evidence of syphilis infection; of 173 homosexuals 67 (39%) tested positive, while among the heterosexuals only 7 out of 49 (14%) tested positive for syphilis.[11]

Another group highly predisposed to acquiring AIDS are intravenous drug abusers. Of almost 9000 cases to date of AIDS in this group, one third are homosexuals and two thirds heterosexuals. The homosexual third, of course, is already at risk for syphilis, but all intravenous drug abusers run an even greater risk of acquiring syphilis, and other venereal diseases, because of the heightened danger of infection via shared needles.[12]

About 23 percent of heterosexual AIDS patients are not also intravenous drug abusers: 1400 cases to date.[13] Of these half are sexual partners of persons with AIDS or at risk of acquiring AIDS. More information is needed on their exposure to venereal disease, but the 1984 CDC study mentioned above found that 2 out of 7 heterosexual patients who were not intravenous drug abusers tested positive for syphilis.[14]

The syphilis connection is often misinterpreted as mere coincidence—due to the fact that persons at risk for AIDS are also at risk for syphilis. A British AIDS researcher, for instance, wrote, "Serological tests for . . . syphilis . . . are frequently positive [in AIDS] *but merely reflect* the high incidence of these infections in the 'at risk' population."[15] Hardly anyone has seriously considered the possibility that preexisting infection with syphilis in this group might be a major cause of AIDS.

One exception was a study performed in Denmark in 1986. The subjects were 100 homosexual-bisexual men being screened for AIDS. Fifty-four had AIDS-virus antibodies, and of this group 36 (63%) had had syphilis. Of the 46 without AIDS antibodies only 16 (35%) had had syphilis. The authors found this to be a statistically significant distinction between the groups. Of the AIDS-virus positive group 12 had had syphilis 4 or 5 times; none in the AIDS-virus negative group had had syphilis as often as three times.

Furthermore, both groups had an equal incidence of gonorrhoea. The authors held that the contrast between the equal incidence of gonorrhoea in the two groups and the unequal incidence of syphilis was "evidence against the supposition that the increased incidence of syphilis among [AIDS-virus] antibody-positive patients merely reflects an increased frequency of sexually transmitted diseases."[16]

In other words, if infection with syphilis merely reflected

the likelihood of picking up this venereal disease while pursuing the gay lifestyle, its incidence should have been identical in the two groups, as was the case for gonorrhoea.

The 1983 CDC study mentioned above—comparing PCP or KS cases with healthy homosexual controls—found much the same relationship between syphilis and gonorrhoea: while almost twice as many KS or PCP cases had had syphilis than controls (68% vs. 36%), the incidence of gonorrhoea was much the same in the two groups (86% vs. 74%).[17]

Thus the relationship between syphilis and AIDS seems to differ from the relationship between gonorrhoea and AIDS.

□ □ □ □ □

A recent survey of 100 male homosexuals in Berkeley, California, by Joan McKenna and coworkers (see Appendix A) found that 24 were diagnosed as having AIDS and that 16 of the 24 showed evidence of syphilis infection. On these and other grounds McKenna concluded that "epidemic syphilis" may be a major factor predisposing to infection with the AIDS virus.[18]

□ □ □ □ □

We maintain that there is a causal connection between AIDS and syphilis and not merely a coincidental one. There are many reasons for believing this aside from those already mentioned.

In the first place, AIDS and AIDS-related conditions often resemble syphilis, leading to diagnostic confusion. A 1984 article on "Secondary Syphilis Masquerading as AIDS in a Young Gay Male" described a 38-year-old white homosexual admitting to over 5000 sexual partners in the previous 16 years. His combination of "constitutional complaints, diffuse lymph node enlargement, and widespread skin lesions was mistakenly attributed to AIDS by both the patient and the medical staff upon admission. Indeed, many of these features were compatible with either the AIDS-related complex, which may represent a prodrome to the development of full-blown AIDS, or with disseminated KS."[19]* Further investigation, however, led to a diagnosis of syphilis.

A 1986 case ultimately diagnosed as secondary meningovascular syphilis was also first taken to be AIDS. The attending physician wrote: "In the Northeast, symptoms of weight loss, generalized lymphadenopathy, fever, and malaise in a young patient with a history of intravenous heroin abuse suggest the diagnosis of AIDS or AIDS-related complex."[20]

□ □ □ □ □

Over 700 persons have acquired AIDS through blood transfusions.[21] But syphilis can also be transmitted via blood transfusion, especially if new blood is used immediately without being stored for a few days.[22] Blood supplies, by the way, are rarely tested for syphilis.[23]

AIDS seems to occur in the newborn. But this is merely a parallel with congenital syphilis, of which there are almost 300 cases a year in the United States—rising from just over 100 cases annually in 1978.[24] Thus congenital syphilis is probably being diagnosed as AIDS.

Several other groups have a high incidence of AIDS, and in all of them a syphilitic background is evident.

In 1982 the disease was reported in the U.S. Haitian community, the great majority of whom denied being homosexuals or drug abusers, and today about 3–5% of cases are Haitians.[25]† But this can readily be explained in terms

---

*"Prodrome" means the symptoms occurring in the very early stages of a disease, or preceding the onset of the disease.

†On April 2, 1985, the CDC eliminated the category of "Haitians" from its reports on incidence of AIDS in the United States. They were incorporated in the category "none of the above" and at the time comprised the whole of that category (*Washington Post* April 9, 1985). The CDC has never given an explanation for this change and denied that political considerations played any role.

of syphilis, as Haiti is perhaps the spot in the Western Hemisphere with the highest incidence of syphilis.

It is largely confined to the Haitian urban population, while yaws—a related treponemal disease spread by sexual contact and which is probably also an AIDS cofactor—has been endemic in the countryside for centuries.

While the statistics are less than reliable (Haiti does not possess a Public Health Service or a Ministry of Health), a 1916 survey of 850 persons chosen at random by U.S. Navy medical personnel found that 74 percent gave a positive Wasserman reaction.[26] As late as 1949 an investigation concluded that almost 5% of the population was infected—a level 28 times that of the United States in that year.[27] A 1983 study of AIDS in Haiti found that 7 out of 31 patients had a previous history of syphilis.[28]

Another area of the world in which AIDS is epidemic is the part of East Africa which includes Ruanda, Uganda, and northeastern Zaire, where it is found almost entirely in a heterosexual population.[29] A recent *Lancet* article described AIDS incidence in Zaire as "comparable with or higher than the rate in San Francisco or New York."[30] Kaposi's Sarcoma is endemic in Ruanda.[31] The *Washington Post* reported in 1986 that AIDS in Uganda is "one of the country's major health problems," that "at least ten percent of the capital's sexually active population is infected with antibodies" to the AIDS virus, and that it is the leading cause of death in the local hospital. The number of new cases was reportedly doubling every six months, and a hospital spokesman called it "a human disaster situation like the eruption of Mt. St. Helen's, like the Mexico City earthquake."[32]

Less well-known is the fact that syphilis has been endemic in these areas for decades. A 1929 survey in Uganda estimated that *eighty percent* of the population had been infected, and a 1966 study found that 15% of the population showed evidence of previous infection.[33] A 1972 article stated, "syphilis is highly prevalent in certain sectors of the population in

Uganda."[34]

Physicians in Zimbabwe reported in 1985 that "syphilis continues to be an important infectious disease in Zimbabwe," and a survey of 200 persons chosen at random in the capital city found 7.5 percent testing positive for syphilis.[35] In Zambia a study found an incidence of 5 percent in males and 10 percent in females.[36] A 1985 survey in the southern Sudan including 1767 subjects found that 35 percent of males, and 38 percent of females, tested positive.[37] A 1987 study in Zaire found that 11 out of 100 healthy controls (11%) tested positive for syphilis, and an editorial in the *Journal of the American Medical Association* noted, "overall, it is clear that many African populations, like certain high-risk groups for [AIDS-virus] infection in the United States, show a higher seroprevalence to certain infectious agents in comparison with heterosexual control groups in non-African populations. Notably, these agents include . . . syphilis."[38]

Not surprisingly, AIDS patients from these countries show a high incidence of syphilis in their background. An investigation of 25 patients in Ruanda, for instance, found that 11 tested positive for syphilis; a study of AIDS patients from Ruanda and Zaire conducted in Belgium found that nearly 10% tested positive for syphilis.[39]

A 1986 study of AIDS in Nairobi prostitutes found that between 24 and 52 percent (depending on the test used) of "low status" ladies of the night had been infected with syphilis; for the "high status" ones, the range was still between 25 and 38 percent.[40] In Ivory Coast almost 74 percent of a sample of prostitutes from the capital were infected with *Treponema pallidum*; for prostitutes in the whole country the figure was 47 percent, and about a quarter of these also manifested AIDS-virus antibodies; prisoners had a 38 percent incidence of *T. pallidum* infection and about a 10 percent incidence of AIDS-virus antibodies; in one town even the hotel staff showed almost a 22 percent incidence of syphilis infection and an 11 percent infection with one or another AIDS virus.[41]

The 1987 study in Zaire mentioned earlier found that 6 out of a group of 38 AIDS patients tested positive for syphilis.[42]

Kaposi's Sarcoma is endemic in the same regions of Africa where syphilis is also widespread, i.e., northeastern Zaire and western Uganda.[43] In the past it was confused with syphilis, and syphilis was part of the differential diagnosis; some authorities saw syphilis as a predisposing cause of KS.[44]

The connection with AIDS is obvious. The situation in Africa, moreover, throws light on AIDS in Haiti. In the 1960's several thousand Haitian professional people migrated to Zaire to fill jobs left by the departing colonial administration; they very probably brought the AIDS virus back with them on returning to Haiti.[45] But no one has yet called attention to the extraordinary incidence of syphilis and yaws in Haiti or suggested these as AIDS cofactors.

□ □ □ □ □

It might be asked why only a proportion of AIDS cases are found to have a syphilis background. If this disease is as important an AIDS cofactor as we maintain, why is the figure not 100 percent in all surveys.

This brings up a problem which has bedevilled syphilis research for many decades — the unreliability of all laboratory tests for the presence or absence of this disease, causing a proliferation of "false positive" or "false negative" results.

In principle, a "positive" outcome means that signs of the disease have been detected. By the same token, a "negative" reading means "no disease." If the individual is free of the disease, but the test states otherwise, that is a "false positive." If the test shows him to be disease-free, whereas he is actually infected, that is a "false negative."

One series of tests looks for the treponeme itself somewhere inside the body. But microscopic examination of fluid from a syphilitic sore ("chancre") for presence of the *T. pallidum* can be vitiated if topical antibiotics have been used on the chancre, since they inactivate the treponemes and may give a "false negative" reading; on the other hand, if fluid is taken from the mouth, rectum, cervix, or vagina for examination, the ordinary microorganisms which live there often cannot be distinguished by their shape from the treponeme — which could lead to a "false positive" result. Or the treponeme may not be discovered; especially in cases of long-term infection, very few are to be found in the circulation, and they may be difficult to detect — again a "false negative."[46]

This "treponemal" test is relatively expensive. Much less costly are the tests, known as "serological," which seek to measure antibodies to the *T. pallidum* in the patient's blood serum. Of these the VDRL ("Venereal Disease Research Laboratory") and the RPR ("rapid plasma reagin") treponemal antibody tests are the best known, being used for large-scale screening. They detect antibodies which are "non-specific," meaning probably provoked by the syphilis treponeme but not necessarily, and can be thrown off in a number of ways. An individual can be "positive" (or "seropositive") as a result of an acute febrile illness, genital herpes, cirrhosis of the liver, infectious mononucleosis, smallpox vaccination, leprosy, autoimmune disease, heroin addiction, and many other factors. Or a false positive reading may be simply congenital.[47]

The VDRL and RPR may yield a false "seronegative" reading, especially at early stages of the disease; in one reported series the VDRL failed to detect reactivity in 57 percent of patients who had been previously infected with *T. pallidum*.[48]

Somewhat more precise is the fluorescent treponemal antibody-absorbed (FTA-ABS) test for treponemal antibody, but it cannot distinguish syphilis from other treponemal diseases, such as yaws. The FTA-ABS becomes positive earlier in the disease than the VDRL. But it can yield a false positive reading if the patient has abnormal immune globulins in the blood due to rheumatoid arthritis or some related disease; pregnancy also sometimes gives rise to a false positive.[49] The margin of error has been found, in various series, to be 7, 10, and even 37 percent.[50]

14

And a person who has been successfully treated for syphilis usually remains FTA-ABS positive for life; thus no laboratory test can determine if he has been reinfected.

Paradoxically, an individual who has had syphilis for many years or decades, and whose body has learned to coexist with it, often tests negative.[51]

There are many other laboratory tests, a situation which has been described as a "serological Tower of Babel."[52] None of them is perfect, and, in general, the more sensitive they are, the greater the likelihood of false positive results. Furthermore, as in any human endeavor, greater precision costs more money, and this money is often not available. The surveys of AIDS patients for a syphilis background are thus full of uncertainties.

Stephen S. Caiazza, M.D., of New York, who treats many AIDS patients and is convinced that the disease is caused by an underlying syphilis (see Appendix B), states that his patients "invariably test negative when the standard tests for syphilis are used, but when more sophisticated ones are employed, such as the FTA and others, the yield approaches 100 percent."

We suspect that if all AIDS patients were given the full battery of serological and treponemal tests for syphilis, the incidence would be found to "approach 100 percent." But the AIDS virus itself may be introducing a factor of confusion. Mary E. Guinan of the Centers for Disease Control suggests that AIDS-virus infection compromises the immune system so that the individual no longer reacts appropriately to therapy.[53] Since many tests for syphilis, especially the serological (non-treponemal) ones, rely on an immune reaction, serious immune-system damage may affect the tests also. Caiazza thinks that the AIDS virus interferes with serological tests and gives as an example a patient who repeatedly tested positive for syphilis and whose reaction disappeared or became extremely weak once he became sick with AIDS.[54] In a January, 1987, letter to the AMA *Journal* (not published) he wrote: "We wish to emphasize the inherent difficulty in making the diagnosis of treponemal infection, especially if a patient also is, or has been, infected with Human Immunodeficiency Virus (HIV) . . . clinicians must be alert . . . to the real difficulty in making the initial diagnosis—especially if there is a concomitant HIV infection."[55] This conclusion was supported by an editorial in the June 18, 1987, *New England Journal of Medicine*, by Edmund C. Tramont, M.D., Chief of Infectious Diseases at the Walter Reed Army Medical Center in Washington, D.C. He stated: (1) the "bedrock for the diagnosis of syphilis" is the serologic test which relies on the patient's antibody response, i.e., on the capacity of the patient's immune system to respond to the test; and (2) "the antibody response in HIV-infected patients, particularly in the later stages of AIDS, may be compromised, and thus the diagnosis may be obscured."[56]

In non-technical language, once the individual with syphilis becomes infected with AIDS-virus, the syphilis may well become impossible to diagnose. Hence certain AIDS patients may test negative for the presence of syphilis even though their clinical features and clinical history demonstrate the contrary.

This very serious diagnostic and epidemiologic problem awaits a solution.

□ □ □ □ □

One of the many puzzling features of the AIDS epidemic has been its peculiar distribution pattern. To date 95 percent of American cases have been in the three categories: male homosexuals (66 percent), intravenous drug abusers who are mostly males and homosexuals (25 percent), and heterosexuals who are not intravenous drug abusers (4 percent). An additional three percent is accounted for by blood transfusions, and the remainder are "undetermined" (this includes the congenital cases, which are equally puzzling). No one has succeeded in explaining this strange pattern of incidence, nor in tying it to the high incidence among heterosexuals in Africa and Haiti.

We maintain that the syphilis connection provides the first plausible explanation of the apparently bizarre distribution of AIDS cases in the world.

3

Syphilis Suppression During the Great Postwar Penicillin Fallout

During "the great penicillin fallout" from 1945 to 1960 physicians noted a startling alteration in the appearance of the typical case of syphilis.[1] The classic symptoms of the disease were appearing much less frequently and were apparently being "masked" or in some way disguised or perverted by the penicillin.

Ordinarily, the first sign of syphilis infection is the chancre — a sore which appears at the site of infection after an incubation period of one to three months and marks the onset of the "primary" stage. Then the adjacent lymph glands become swollen and rubbery, a condition known as "regional lymphadenopathy."

Thereafter the disease "matures" for up to six months and enters the "secondary" stage, characterized by a "macular" (spotty) roseola-like rash and other skin symptoms. The regional lymphadenopathy becomes generalized and affects the body's whole lymphatic system; it is a "valuable diagnostic finding" and "one of the most characteristic aspects" of syphilis; the lymph nodes are "painless," "enlarged, rubbery, non-tender, and freely movable."[2]

The patient will complain of rashes, fever, itching, sore

throat, headache, malaise, vertigo, sweating, insomnia, nausea, prostration, weight loss, loss of hair, or aching in the bones and joints. Some have hypertension, kidney disease, swollen liver, or swollen spleen; others have a subacute meningitis with cranial nerve involvement. In this stage syphilis is often confused with such conditions as infectious mononucleosis, iritis, neuroretinitis, lichen planus, cancer, nephritis, dementia, lymphomas, psoriasis and other skin eruptions, and even drug reactions. For this reason secondary syphilis is called "the great imitator."[3]

If the primary or secondary stages are not treated at all, or are treated inadequately, two-thirds of the time the symptoms will disappear, the patient will feel better, and no trace of the treponeme can be found in his fluids or solids. This is called the "early latent" stage. *However, he is still infectious,* since the disease can relapse back into the secondary stage; such relapses, in fact, occur in from 1 to 5 percent of patients and are a natural part of the disease process.[4]

The patient who is treated successfully during the primary or secondary stages, i.e., "cured" of syphilis, cannot readily be distinguished from the one whose disease is in the latent stage.[5] The principal difference between them is that the patient in the early latent period is still infectious.

After some months or years the patient enters the "late latent stage," when relapse is, in principle, no longer possible, or at least unlikely. But there is no uniform line of demarcation between the "early" and "late" latent stages. A handbook on syphilis published in 1961 by the U.S. Public Health Service could only "suggest" that the "great majority" of cases enter the late latent stage within two years after the infection and "probably," "for epidemiologic purposes," the first year is the most infectious.[6] Other authorities estimate that, regardless of treatment, the patient remains infectious for up to four years.[7]

A woman who has been "cured" of syphilis can convey it to her fetus throughout her whole childbearing period![8]

After the latent stage comes tertiary syphilis, when the treponeme penetrates the brain and nervous system and causes neurological disorders.[9]

□ □ □ □ □

During the post-war decades the saturation of American society with penicillin did not spare syphilis. It too was treated more or less indiscriminately first with penicillin and later with newer antibiotics. Furthermore, many cases were treated inadvertently when patients took prescriptions for other conditions. The outcome was often a "masking" or "disguising" of the primary and secondary symptoms, with the disease seemingly entering the latent stage at the very outset.

Physicians at this time debated extensively whether syphilis was actually being "cured." The chancre sometimes healed over as a result of antibiotics, while the patient remained diseased and infectious. Furthermore, as noted by the 1961 Public Health Service handbook, antibiotic use "altered serologic patterns in many cases without effecting complete cures".[10] The *New England Journal of Medicine* editorialized in 1951, "The small doses of penicillin used in the treatment of gonorrhoea may modify an initial lesion of syphilis, or even prevent its occurrence without producing its complete cure".[11]

The unanswered question was how often this was occurring. Syphilis had long been known to occur frequently in a nonsymptomatic form. A 1947 textbook stated, "from 25 to 40 percent of syphilis is acquired without recognition by the patient of lesions, i.e., without chancre or rash. This is more frequent in women."[12] A 1958 textbook on bacterial diseases observed:

> The control of syphilis is made particularly difficult because many infected individuals are not aware that they have the disease; this is particularly the case in females in whom the early lesions may be entirely within the genital tract and largely symptomless.[13]

The outcome was that many people, perhaps women in particular, became infected with syphilis without ever realizing it! The mild postwar syphilis was made even milder by the penicillin fallout. Researchers at Johns Hopkins in 1952 speculated that "entirely symptomless syphilitic infection as a result of penicillin alone is an uncommon occurrence," but other physicians in these years assumed that this sort of "arrested syphilis" was rather common.[14] Some were cured, others were not; "happenstance" treatment with antibiotics merely confused the clinical picture, so that neither the physician nor the patient himself had a true idea of what was actually going on.[15]

□ □ □ □ □

Curing syphilis, even with antibiotics, required more skill than was at this time possessed by the ordinary GP, armed with nothing more than "a syringe and a bottle of penicillin." Penicillin acts on the treponeme only in the stage of replication and is maximally effective when administered immediately after infection in the primary stage of the disease. At that time the treponemes are readily accessible to the action of penicillin and are usually disposed of rather quickly.*

However, the treponeme spreads rapidly through the body within a short time after infection and eventually makes its way through the "blood-brain barrier" into the cerebrospinal fluid, the eyeball, and other recesses where it ceases replication altogether or replicates very slowly, thus becoming relatively invulnerable to the medicine's action (the benzathine

---

*They are entirely resistant in the non-replicating stage and can readily be maintained for long periods in a penicillin solution. One physician wrote: "Anyone who has watched the spirochete of syphilis moving actively in a concentrated solution of penicillin for hours under the microscope cannot help being impressed with the importance of the time factor in destroying the organism" (Armand J. Pereyra *et al.*, "A Graphic Guide for Clinical Management of Latent Syphilis." *California Medicine* 112:5 [May, 1970], 13–18).

penicillin used today cannot "penetrate the blood-brain barrier").[16] Latent and tertiary (neuro-) syphilis are much more difficult to treat with success, since by this time the treponemes have found refuge in inaccessible cracks and crannies of the body.[17]

And, although the treponeme is usually found extracellularly, it can also penetrate tissue cells and live inside them, where it is protected from the penicillin; perhaps this is why ocular and neurosyphilis can continue to progress clinically even when no treponemes are detectable in the patient's body.[18]

Of course, the AIDS virus is also known to be capable of penetrating lymphocytes and other cells and living there sheltered from the action of most kinds of drug therapy.[19]

The successful cure of syphilis requires a close understanding of the disease process in the specific patient. Various standardized treatments have been proposed: today it is 2.4 million units of penicillin G benzathine given intramuscularly in one dose.[20] But individualization is a necessity. Even the most skillful treatment is not uniformly successful. Failure rates in primary or secondary syphilis are thought to range from 4 percent after one year to 11 percent after two years.[22] Failure rates in tertiary syphilis are also estimated at about 10 percent.[23]

Treponemes have been found safe and sound in the patient's body, even after 100 million units of penicillin therapy.[24] Facts such as this led one author to comment, "of all bacteria, *Treponema pallidum* is at the same time one of the most sensitive and most resistant germs to the action of penicillin."[25] A medical school professor wrote in 1971: "These reports challenge the long cherished belief that properly administered penicillin is unfailingly effective therapy for syphilis, and have also raised new questions about the host-parasite relations in late syphilis."[24]

Because serological and treponemal test results are often so misleading, successful treatment can be verified only by tracking all the patient's sexual contacts to ascertain if they have been infected by him. But this is so difficult, expensive, and tedious that it is rarely done. Allocating public health officers to this time-consuming task is expensive.* And the close supervision of patients and their contacts is rendered more difficult by the mobility of American society. Hence the data are gathered very imperfectly.

An authority on public health aspects of syphilis wrote in 1964:

> Great effort is expended to trace down all known and suspected cases of syphilis, but, as every experienced epidemiologist knows, it is an endless task . . . an able venereal disease investigator traced the chain of infection started by a sixteen-year-old boy named Victor. Some 96 teenagers are interviewed. Of these, 18 are found to have syphilis. Undoubtedly many others have been spared the disease because of prompt apprehension and treatment of these early infectious cases. After almost three months of dedicated effort, the public health worker dares to hope that he may soon reach the end of the trail. Not so, for with dramatic suddenness the track leads back to Victor! Ironically, the chain of infection he started has twisted around to reinfect him. And already he has exposed five new contacts.[27]

The author concluded that this process was an exercise in futility.

---

*A former Public Health Service case officer has told this writer that in the early 1960's he held the New York City record for tracking down sexual contacts of individuals with primary and secondary syphilis — 13 in one month!! This shows how expensive the process is. And no attempt was made to detect the sexual contacts of individuals with latent syphilis whether or not infectious.

The situation has not changed at all in the past twenty years. In 1987 the AMA *Journal* editorialized:

> The treatment of syphilis is still controversial . . . Unfortunately, not enough data are available to determine whether the recommended treatments are optimally effective, or whether the efficacy of these regimens is stable . . . Long intervals may exist between treatment and the determination of therapeutic outcome. The patient may present for only one or two followup visits or may not present at all, making it impossible to determine definitive cure. Therefore, many difficulties exist when attempting to document the overall cure rate for syphilis treatment. Because of the complexity of determining therapeutic cure of syphilis, *no information on temporal trends for treatment failures is available . . . In early studies the failure rates ranged from 0% to 7%. Unfortunately, no recent studies have been done to reassure us that this regimen is equally effective at the present time.* [stress added][28]

But when syphilis is improperly or inadequately treated, the consequences can be unexpected and dismaying. In the 1950's and 1960's the primary and secondary cases declined, but there was an increase in the number of latent ones which were a fertile source of later disease — including AIDS.

The Danish study mentioned earlier, which found that homosexuals testing positive for the AIDS virus had a much higher background incidence of syphilis than those testing negative, found, furthermore, that the "positive" group also had a quite different pattern of syphilis: 29 percent primary, 43 percent secondary, and 37 percent latent. The "negative" group had 52 percent primary, 39 percent secondary, and only 9 percent latent.[29] This higher proportion of latent cases in the AIDS-positive group suggests, of course, that as syphilis progresses into the latent stage, it predisposes to infection with AIDS.

The rise in latent cases was noted by many observers. A director of the New York City Health Department wrote in 1958:

> The failure of the so-called late latent form to decline causes speculation. This form of the disease is recognizable only by the presence of a persistent serologic reaction. It appears paradoxical that the forms of the disease which produce symptoms should decline while the type dependent upon an empirical serum reaction should remain stationary.[30]

Two California physicians warned in 1968:

> Recent clinical experience suggests that the manifestations of early secondary syphilis are becoming fewer and milder. Numerous cases of secondary syphilis are now being seen with a few cutaneous manifestations or an atypical appearance. In the absence of characteristic skin lesions, early secondary syphilis may become manifest as a bizarre syndrome, or it may mimic many systemic diseases.[31]

Another California physician complained in 1970:

> The advent of treponemal antibiotics has shifted the concern of the physician from treatment to diagnosis. Indications are that, far from eradicating syphilis, these antibiotics are driving the disease underground and increasing the difficulty of detection. Although the incidence of the disease has more than trebled since 1955, the chancre and the secondary rash no longer are commonly seen. Undoubtedly some of these lesions are being suppressed, and the disease masked by the indiscriminate use of antibiotics. It is difficult other-

wise to explain the predominance of latent syphilis in current medical practice. *The ominous prospect of a widespread resurgence of the disease in its tertiary form looms ahead.* [stress added][32]

Two French physicians observed in 1983:

It is wrong to assert that a serum level of 0.03 U/ml of penicillin kills all *Treponema pallidum*. Setting up a standard treatment generalized on such reasoning appears to be dangerous when we know that the arguments are quite wrong and that we do not have any criterion of bacteriological sterilization. Thus a standard uniform dosage of penicillin . . . may help to heal superficially a chancre or to remove roseola, but certainly does not give a bacteriologic sterilization in 100% of cases of those who have been invaded by *Treponema pallidum* . . . . It is therefore absolutely essential to undertake treatment at high doses and for a long time to avoid a latent infection which is likely to be the cause of future serious relapses.[33]

An inability to tell if a case was primary, secondary, early latent, late latent, or cured confused the epidemiology of syphilis to the point of unintelligibility. This made a true record of its prevalence in American society even more difficult to obtain which, in turn, has complicated any discussion of its relationship to AIDS.

Syphilis is difficult to detect in a modern society; it carries a heavy stigma, inhibiting reporting and even recognition by the patient himself. Various investigations have shown that private physicians in the United States treat 80 percent of patients with infectious syphilis but only report 10 to 25 percent of these cases to health authorities. The statistics of incidence are thus based on information from the 20% treated in public health clinics and the portion of cases which private physicians choose to report.[34]

Thus, during the decade, 1972–1982, there may have been 50,000 to 100,000 new cases a year in the United States, instead of the 20–30,000 actually reported.[35]

Often enough the physician himself fails to diagnose syphilis in the patient before him. When today's doctors were in medical school, this disease was thought to be on its way out. Hence they received little training in its recognition and treatment and were unprepared for the contemporary increase in cases. The Public Health Service handbook states: "Unfortunately, the revolution in syphilis management occurred during the period when the fewest syphilitics were being seen by the general practitioner; and now the increasing case load is coming upon him when he has been least prepared, and is confronting him with problems which sometimes seem to call for the judgment of Solomon."[36]

And an incidence of even 100,000 new cases yearly comes to less than one case for each practicing physician; so the average doctor has very little experience with it.[37]

The patient with late latent syphilis and positive serology might become reinfected or have a relapse, manifesting few or no signs of the primary chancre or secondary stage and continuing to react positively to serological tests; the physician in that case assumes that the test results are holdovers from the earlier infection and overlooks his infectiousness. This kind of situation is particularly dangerous from the epidemiological standpoint.[38]

In any case, syphilis is no longer a disease of the past. The inescapable conclusion is that there is a great deal of undiagnosed, semi-treated or untreated, infectious latent and not-so-latent syphilis in the U.S. population.

A physician echoed much professional opinion when he wrote in 1983:

Although our concepts of the nature of the sexually transmitted diseases in promiscuous populations have changed during the past decade, and although much attention has been drawn to the newly emerging disorders, the older, typical venereal diseases are still prevalent.[39]

□ □ □ □ □

This diagnostic and epidemiological confusion is especially regrettable in a disease known as "the great imitator." Secondary syphilis can be, and has been, confused diagnostically with an enormous number of medical conditions: acute meningitis, neural hearing loss, iritis, uveitis, optic neuritis, Bell's palsy, numerous gastrointestinal and skin disorders, proctitis, hepatitis, pneumonia, liver or kidney failure, ostitis, arthritis, various cancers, lymphomas, and other malignancies, psoriasis, infectious mononucleosis, mental illness, and many others.[40]

A 1981 survey of 34 patients with secondary syphilis treated in a Detroit public health clinic found that only 14 of the 36 private physicians who had seen these patients earlier had given syphilis as the primary diagnosis; 5 others had included it in the differential diagnosis; 12 had not considered syphilis at all but discovered it later in consequence of a routine serological test; 5 other physicians failed to include syphilis in the diagnosis and did not order serological tests.[41]

It can be assumed that many cases of syphilis are being systematically given wrong diagnostic labels in American medical practice, which may, in turn, confuse the relationship with AIDS. For example, when researchers report, in a series of cases, "an unusually high frequency of infectious mononucleosis years before the onset of the [AIDS] syndrome," one wonders if syphilis has not been overlooked.[42]

Quite recently, as this book was going to press, two articles appeared which discussed in graphic detail the possibility of confusion between syphilis and AIDS and showed how great the overlap between them can be.

C. D. Berry, M.D. and coauthors described a patient with

both secondary syphilis and AIDS-virus infection who was treated with benzathine penicillin but relapsed after five months into tertiary (neuro-) syphilis. They comment: "the role of HIV infection and its associated immunocompromised conditions in relapse of syphilis is unknown . . . [but] the immunological abnormalities associated with HIV infection may permit more treponemal proliferation and dissemination than occur in immunologically intact hosts. . . . Further studies are required . . . [on] the efficacy of currently recommended therapy, since benzathine penicillin does not achieve treponemicidal levels in the central nervous system; and [on] the possible effect of HIV infection on the progression of syphilis and the response to therapy."[43]

The second article, by Donald R. Johns and coauthors, described four cases of neurosyphilis in young homosexual men with serologic evidence of AIDS-virus infection. Two of them had undergone adequate benzathine penicillin therapy for early syphilis. In one of them the neurosyphilis developed *within four months after the primary infection,* "consistent with an accelerated course of syphilitic infection." They conclude that the *T. pallidum* and the AIDS virus can interact in two principal ways:

—the immune collapse caused by the AIDS virus may suppress the individual's response to infection with syphilis, causing a more rapid progress of the latter disease.
—*immune-suppression caused by syphilis may have a similar effect on host defenses against AIDS.*[44]

Both of these mechanisms are real possibilities. The AIDS-virus-infected individual may become infected with syphilis, which then follows an accelerated course (see Appendix B). Or the *T. pallidum*-infected individual becomes infected with AIDS-virus. In our opinion, the first of these mechanisms is relatively rare today but will become more and more common in the future, as persons infected with AIDS virus become exposed to syphilis. The second mechanism is, without doubt, the most common today, as our centuries of contact with syphilis make us vulnerable to this AIDS virus which was once probably innocuous but has now become lethal.

4

Syphilis
and the Immune System

This subterranean pool, or swamp, of undiagnosed and untreated or semitreated syphilis is significant for the emergence of AIDS because syphilis is an immunosuppressive disease. Especially in the early stages the *T. pallidum* can suspend or inactivate the body's system of immune protection.[1]

Those who harbor syphilis unknowingly for extended periods of time are slowly undermining their capacity to withstand other infections. The outcome is the state of immune collapse which we call "acquired immune-deficiency syndrome"—*acquired from syphilis.*

□ □ □ □ □

The healthy human body has two interlocking systems of immune protection—"humoral" and "cellular." Humoral immunity is produced by elements found in the blood and other fluids, specifically antibodies and other "immune globulins." Cellular immunity, on the other hand, is the task of the bone marrow and the thymus. The former produces bits of protein called lymphocytes, a part of which then pass through the thymus gland to become "thymus" or "T" lymphocytes.

These come in several sizes and shapes, and with different functions. Subsets—such as the "T-helper cells," "T-suppressor cells," and "T-killer cells"—perform different roles in producing immunity. The T-helper cells help stimulate the production of antibodies and assist other components of the body's system of immune defense. The T-suppressor cells act as a negative feedback to turn off or suppress the immunologic response once the danger to the host has passed; if there are too many, or if they are too active, the immune response will be deadened. In the normal, non-immune-deficient individual there should be up to twice as many T-helper as T-suppressor cells.

The *Treponema pallidum* acts specifically against the thymus gland.[2] The thymus-dependent parts of the lymphatic system deteriorate, and there is consequent decrease in the numbers of T-lymphocytes.[3] The T-helper cells are particularly affected by this: there is a decline in their number and the ratio with the T-suppressor cells is reversed.[4] Consequently, a long-term effect of syphilis is loss of, or decline in, the system of immunity, and a lowering of the individual's capacity to defend himself against other infectious conditions.[5] In this respect, of course, it resembles AIDS. Stephen Caiazza states: "Like AIDS it makes the individual vulnerable to a host of opportunistic infections which a healthy person would easily ward off."

In laboratory experiments the blood and serum from patients with primary and secondary syphilis have repeatedly been demonstrated to possess immunosuppressive properties.[6]

Thus a major cause of the present AIDS epidemic has undoubtedly been the "masking" of syphilis by antibiotic abuse, suppressing the disease and causing it to smolder away for decades like an underground fire. It has slowly burned out the immune systems of a large proportion of those who have been treated for syphilis with antibiotics—knowingly or unknowingly—since 1945. This opened the door to a virus which may be quite new or, on the contrary, may for centuries have occupied an inconspicuous niche in the order of nature until brought to life by the new opportunities.

□ □ □ □ □

The syphilitic background of AIDS is seen from the symptomatic and other parallels between the two conditions.

The first is lymphadenopathy. As already noted, this is "one of the most characteristic symptoms" of syphilis. General lymphadenopathy and enlargement of the spleen are also very characteristic features of the AIDS syndrome. Typically, a history of "progressive generalized lymphadenopathy antedates AIDS by about 18 months."[7]

The AIDS outbreak in San Francisco was preceded by an epidemic of generalized lymphadenopathy which started in 1979 and lasted several years. Physicians explained it as activation of the immune system, "most likely from having too many sexual partners and too many sexually transmitted diseases, and from using too many recreational drugs."[8] The lymph nodes are "most often described as nontender." Among the swollen lymph nodes in these patients were ones found most particularly in secondary syphilis!![9]

In 1984 a survey was made of 200 U.S. males with the lymphadenopathy syndrome: 90 percent had had gonorrhoea, while 70 percent had been treated for warts in the genital area (often of venereal origin). The authors noted that "they have past histories of multiple sexually transmitted diseases," especially syphilis and hepatitis, and that some had tested positive on one of the standard syphilis blood tests, "which clearly indicates what might be the cause of their lymphadenopathy."[10] If the tests had been done with meticulous care, probably all of these men would have been found to be infected with syphilis.

The authors described two cases of the 200 who "transformed" to AIDS. The first was a 31-year-old man with a positive serologic test for syphilis. The second was a 34-year-old man who developed AIDS together with a non-healing cancerous rectal fissure and a type of meningitis (all findings suggestive of syphilis).[11]

The "AIDS-related complex" (ARC), a milder version which may or may not develop into AIDS, also involves swollen lymph nodes.

□ □ □ □ □

In the second place, AIDS is marked by deterioration, destruction, or collapse of the thymus and a decline in the numbers of T-lymphocytes.[12] A National Institutes of Health researcher stated in 1985 that the AIDS virus "turns the T-cell off from being a lymphocyte and on to being a AIDS-virus factory."[13] The ordinary ratio of 1:1 or 2:1 between T-helper and T-suppressor cells drops to 1:2 or lower.[14] The immune system lapses into neutrality and opens the body to invasion by a host of ordinarily "commensal" microorganisms.*

In the late 1970's and early 1980's several studies of American homosexual men showed them to be suffering from a reversal in the ratio of T-helper to T-suppressor cells, even when appearing perfectly healthy and manifesting no signs of disease.[15] Lymphadenopathy was often a part of the overall syndrome. One study suggested that the T-cell reversal was due to their use of amyl nitrite inhalents but went on to state: "The very high prevalence of immunological abnormalities among homosexual men suggests that as yet unidentified host and environmental characteristics may contribute . . . . Further study is needed to disentangle the roles of amyl nitrites, viruses, and other factors in the development of immunodeficiency . . . ." The authors noted that the test subjects had a "history of hepatitis and syphilis" but did not give details.[16]

□ □ □ □ □

---

*This term, meaning "eating at the same table," was coined by Rene Dubos to characterize the bacteria and viruses which usually live in peace with the host. The ordinary healthy human being has *two pounds* of such commensal microorganisms within the gastrointestinal tract and on the surface of the body.

Another parallel between AIDS and syphilis is the overlap among the many symptoms of the two conditions. Acute AIDS infection is known to present with a spotty "roseola-like rash," and a group of Danish researchers in 1986 suggested that "the characteristic skin eruption, which mimics roseola, may be a dermatological marker of acute [AIDS] infection."[17] Of course a roseola-like rash is a major sign of secondary syphilis.

But AIDS predisposes to an enormous variety of different infections and diseases, being as much an "imitator" as secondary syphilis itself. "Indeed," Caiazza states, "there is no clinical sign or symptom associated with AIDS that has not already been reported in the syphilis literature!"

Almost any one can be found: sore throat, hoarseness, fever, night-sweats, headaches, malaise, flu-like symptoms, meningitis-like symptoms, loss of appetite, weight loss, various cutaneous lesions, hair loss, intestinal troubles and lesions, enlarged spleen, kidney troubles, hearing loss, blindness, musculo-skeletal aching; candida, herpes simplex, cytomegalovirus and other infections; hepatitis, tuberculosis, various kinds of pneumonia including *Pneumocystis carinii* pneumonia, and Kaposi's Sarcoma.[18]

In 1985 the AIDS virus was found to be able to "seed the brains" of individuals who might escape immediate damage to the immune system, only to come down later with meningitis, dementia, and various other infections and disorders of the brain and central nervous system.[19] This last group of conditions is, of course, reminiscent of tertiary syphilis which also takes a neurological form.

In another parallel, both AIDS and syphilis seem to affect the male more than the female; in all categories of both diseases males predominate by far.[20]

The ability of the AIDS virus to remain dormant for years, while the "carrier" himself is infectious to others, is also reminiscent of the latent stage in syphilis.[21]

□ □ □ □ □

No one dies of AIDS itself, but the collapsed immune system predisposes to infection with whatever are the common diseases of the time and place. Thus there are striking differences between the typical case of AIDS in the United States and in Africa or Haiti.

The two conditions most frequently associated today with AIDS in the United States are *Pneumocystis carinii* pneumonia and Kaposi's Sarcoma. Both have been historically associated with syphilis and also with immune collapse.

The *Pneumocystis carinii* microorganism has been known to science since the early twentieth century. The lung inflammation which it caused was classified as one of the "atypical," "plasma cell," or "interstitial" pneumonias.[22] It was called "atypical" because it failed to respond to penicillin or sulfonamide therapy, although it seemed to yield to aureomycin and other medicines of this class.[23]

This disease was considered mild, even in children; the death rate was extremely low, being described by one author as "practically nil."[24]

It had been pointed out, however, that PCP was more serious in those with defective immune systems or lowered immune defenses from whatever cause—such as protein malnutrition—explaining why it was more serious in children or adults debilitated by other diseases.[25] This warning took on particular relevance in 1968 when the pneumonia struck a group of 19 children with cancer who were being given immunosuppressive drugs in a children's hospital in Tennessee.[26]

PCP in this decade became fused with pneumonia of syphilitic origin.[27] Syphilis in the past had been known as a cause of pneumonia.[28] The "white lung" which is characteristic of syphilitic pneumonia is often found in the PCP patient,[29] while cases diagnosed as syphilis were turning up with the same "white lung."[30] It was noted that this condition could be confused diagnostically with PCP.[31]

In 1976 scientists at the CDC laboratories in Atlanta were puzzled by the deaths of two owl monkeys and two chimpanzees from PCP infection. This was the first recorded death of a monkey from this disease, and the scientists could not determine the source of the infection. One of the owl monkeys had been experimentally inoculated with *T. pallidum* three years earlier, but the significance of this fact was not appreciated at the time.[32]

In the 1970's Kaposi's Sarcoma first started appearing in Americans with disabled immune function. In 1981 it was reported to be spreading in this country among young homosexual or bisexual males, and the same aggressive form appeared at the same time in Africa.[33] The patients were immunosuppressed, and had depressed levels of T-helper lymphocytes.

As we have noted earlier, both PCP and KS are often found in association with syphilis.[34]

By 1982 both KS and PCP were for the first time occurring in the same individual, and also in conjunction with AIDS, with a mortality rate of up to 68 percent.[35]

In their symptomatology and pathology both PCP and KS resemble the protean manifestations of primary and secondary syphilis but in somewhat different ways. Both have such general symptoms as chills, fever, malaise, weight loss, and anemia; both have many pulmonary symptoms, such as shortness of breath, bronchopneumonia, cough, and emphysema; both have cardiovascular symptoms, lymphadenopathy, muscle pains, and edema, as well as pharyngitis, enlarged spleen, thrush, diarrhoea, and gastritis. But KS has several other sets of associated symptoms: hepatitis, visceral lesions and plaques (rubbery protuberances, also known as gummata) on the skin and lungs as well as kidney symptoms and many more skin manifestations than PCP. The more specific features of KS indicating kinship with syphilis are: purple lesions on the earlobe, infiltrating interstitial pneumonia of the lungs, gummata of the lungs, sarcoid-like granulomas, and strawberry-like facial lesions.[36]

In Africa and Haiti, the most common AIDS symptoms

are gastrointestinal and dermatologic, profound weight loss, fever, diarrhoea, cough, loss of appetite, difficult breathing, and pruritus.[37] Oral and other candida infections occur in half the patients. Other associated conditions are: loss of appetite, skin eruptions, central nervous system infections, tuberculosis, meningitis, and herpes virus infection.[38] In Haiti and in African patients treated in Europe, a very common form of AIDS is disseminated toxoplasmosis (infection with the *Toxoplasma* microorganism).[39]

The lymphadenopathy which is so common in the United States is seen in only 11 percent of African patients.[40] Kaposi's Sarcoma is found very frequently in both groups of patients. Whereas over 60 percent of American patients die from PCP pneumonia, this is found in only 14 percent of African patients treated in Europe.[41]

What is common to all cases, however, is that the diseases associated with AIDS are caused by bacteria and viruses found in healthy persons and which become malignant because of the patient's depressed immune system.[42] One group of researchers notes, "It is possible that patients living in tropical areas and immunosuppressed as a result of [AIDS virus] will manifest other infections endemic in these areas, such as leishmaniasis, leprosy, malaria, filariasis, and other parasitic and bacterial infections."[43]

☐ ☐ ☐ ☐ ☐

The possibility of this sort of immune depression has not been overlooked, but, while numerous diseases have been proposed for this immunosuppressive role, syphilis has been left out of consideration.* Cytomegalovirus infection (found in 95 percent

---

*Of particular interest is Joseph A. Sonnabend *et al.*, "A Multifactorial Model for the Development of AIDS in Homosexual Men," *Annals of the New York Academy of Sciences* 437 (1984), 177–183, which concentrates on the Epstein-Barr virus and cytomegalovirus but ignores syphilis altogether. See, also, Joseph Sonnabend *et al.*, "Acquired Immunodeficiency Syndrome, Opportunistic Infections,

of homosexual men, often in the semen), Hepatitis B, and Epstein-Barr virus infections all have immunosuppressive capacities.[44] For that matter, human semen itself is immuno-suppressive when it passes into the bloodstream, as may happen during anal intercourse with its bruising and laceration of the surrounding tissues.[45] Another immunosuppressive factor, as already mentioned, is use of the amyl nitrite inhalents favored by homosexuals to enhance sexual sensitivity.

But, while these johnny-come-latelies may well make a contribution to AIDS, the protean disease which stands behind all of them — and which is undoubtedly far more immunosuppressive in its nature — has been quite ignored.

This should not be. Syphilis must be far more important as a predisposing factor. It is no accident that this disease has played such a redoubtable role in history. By its intrinsic virulence, its resourcefulness, its adaptability, and its resistance to medication, syphilis has assumed a place in history equal to such other historic scourges of mankind as the bubonic plague, smallpox, tuberculosis, or Asiatic cholera.

If it is being ignored, this is probably for psychological or socio-economic reasons. Having proclaimed the eradication, or at least the taming, of this disease, the medical profession may not want to admit that it was wrong. Furthermore, researchers avid for Nobel prizes may be repelled by the prospect of having once again to tackle the intractable problem of syphilis instead of pursuing some glamorous new virus from an exotic African country. Research funding may be less easy to obtain once AIDS is found to be essentially the reincarnation of syphilis.

Far from being eradicated, however, this disease merely stepped back a pace in order later to spring forward once again. It threatens to wreak as much damage today as ever before in its history, and the sixteenth-century prediction of

---

and Malignancies in Male Homosexuals. A Hypothesis of Etiologic Factors in Pathogenesis." *JAMA* 249:17 (1983), 2370–2374.

Girolamo Fracastoro, the author of the first book on syphilis, is becoming a reality:

> And this disease of which I speak, this syphilis, too, will pass away and die out, but later it will be born again and be seen again by our descendants just as in bygone ages we must believe it was observed by our ancestors.

5

Medicinal
Suppression

But these various diseases are not the only immunosuppressants to which the typical AIDS patient is exposed. The immune system can also be disabled by the cure.

Scant attention has been directed to this aspect of the drugs used in the day-to-day treatment of syphilis and other venereal diseases. But when these medicines are investigated, they are often found to be as harmful to the immune system as the diseases they are used to treat..

Thus medicinal drugs make their contribution to the sustained assault on the immune system which culminates in AIDS.

□ □ □ □ □

Although much has been written in recent years about the "side effects" of drugs used in modern medical practice, this outpouring of knowledge has largely bypassed the immune system. But the physiology of the living organism is a seamless web, with what is called the "immune system" indissolubly connected with every other aspect of the organism's functioning. Any "adverse reaction" will have an impact on the body's ability to muster its immune defenses.

Thus we must acknowledge that our knowledge of the immunodestructive potential of modern medicines is still largely an unwritten chapter. We must always be aware of the extent of our ignorance.

Some evidence, however, has already come to light indicating two types of adverse reactions commonly found in today's medicinal drugs which directly impact on the immune system.

The first relates to the bone marrow and the production of blood components there.

The bone marrow is the organ which produces leucocytes (white blood cells), lymphocytes, eosinophils, monocytes, granulocytes, neutrophils, thrombocytes, and many other components of the blood. Their interrelations are complex, unclear, and, in any case, outside this discussion. What is important is that all issue one way or another from the bone marrow, and all play a role in the body's system of immune defense. Any drug which impairs the creation and functioning of these blood components is thereby impairing the body's immune defenses.

As already noted, the lymphocytes, in particular, play a major role in both AIDS and syphilis and, not unexpectedly, are often implicated in the immunosuppressive effects of drugs.

The second set of adverse reactions which are meaningful for the immune response are those known as allergic, hypersensitivity, or anaphylactic responses — even though their precise relation to changes in the immune system may not always be possible to trace.

Any drug capable of modifying the production of blood-components by the bone marrow, thus of altering the composition of the blood, or of causing an allergic or hypersensitivity reaction, is impairing the immune system.

Most of the medicines used to treat syphilis and other venereal diseases have been implicated in one or both of these adverse reactions affecting the immune system.*

For the treatment of syphilis penicillin is still the most highly recommended drug.[1] The *T. pallidum* does not seem to have become resistant to it, although Mary E. Guinan recently alluded to this possibility and admitted that the truth is not known.[2]

Penicillin has a variety of deleterious effects on the immune system. It is known to lower the content of leucocytes, granulocytes, and neutrophils in the blood, and increase the levels of eosinophils; it can impair the blood-clotting mechanism, causing hemorrhage; occasionally there is hemolytic anemia. Furthermore, the bone marrow may be depressed or cease to mature during penicillin therapy, indicating a direct impact there.[3] Its most pronounced effect, though, is in the realm of allergy. The whole penicillin group causes a very high incidence of allergic and anaphylactic reactions, various studies indicating an incidence of up to 10 percent.[4] These allergic reactions range from death due to anaphylactic shock (in 1 out of 50,000 persons treated with penicillin) to a series of lesser reactions: skin rashes of all types, urticaria, contact dermatitis, exfoliative dermatitis, swelling of the face and other parts of the body, giant hives, asthma, chills and fever, arthritis and arthralgia, swollen lymph glands, enlarged spleen, abnormalities of the heart rhythm, kidney damage, blood or albumen in the urine, and mental changes.[5]

Since the penicillin molecule is very small, and very small molecules are generally incapable of provoking hypersensitization, the mechanism of allergy and hypersensitivity is thought

---

*The immunosuppressive effects of drugs are discussed in detail in the various editions of the *Physician's Desk Reference* and in such standard texts as the *Merck Manual*, Eric W. Martin, *Hazards of Medication* (Second Edition. Philadelphia: Lippincott, 1978), and A. G. Gilman, L. S. Goodman, and A. Gilman, eds., *The Pharmaceutical Basis of Therapeutics* (Sixth and Seventh Editions. New York: Macmillan, 1980, 1985). See, also, the *National Disease and Therapeutic Index (NDTI)* (Ambler, Pa.: IMS America, 1986).

to involve breakdown products of penicillin in the body; they form larger-size molecules which subsequently combine with the body's own proteins to form allergenic combinations (known as "haptens").[6]

Tetracycline is the backup medicine for syphilis in those who are penicillin-allergic.[7] But the members of this family — doxycycline (*Vibramycin, Vibra-Tabs*), minocycline (*Minocin*), oxytetracycline (*Terramycin*) — have perhaps an even larger array of immune-system adverse reactions than penicillin. They impair the development of granulocytes, thrombocytes, and lymphocytes and lead to the generation of atypical ones; they suppress the action of phagocytes, cause a plethora of leucocytes, and in general modify the production of blood components. Tetracycline is deposited in the bones and can depress bone maturation in premature infants treated with it.[8]

Like penicillin, it also causes a variety of rashes, urticarias, exfoliative dermatitis and other skin reactions, as well as swelling of the arteries, asthma, and anaphylactic shock.[9]

The third medicine used for syphilis is erythromycin (*Erytab, E.E.S., E-mycin*, etc.). This is generally thought to be a mild medicine, with a minimum of adverse reactions. However, it also is capable of suppressing lymphocyte function and increasing the numbers of eosinophils in the blood, as well as causing allergic reactions, urticaria and other skin eruptions, liver dysfunction, and anaphylactic shock.[10]

Thus all three of the major drugs used in treating syphilis themselves have immunosuppressive potential.

□ □ □ □ □

But in tracking the genesis of AIDS we are interested in the whole way of life of those who are particularly vulnerable. Joan McKenna and her coworkers in Berkeley, California, described as follows the medical histories of a group of 100 homosexual men interviewed by them:

Among the most common presentations we have found

are the following:

Gonorrhoea: multiple incidents with treatment by antibiotic therapies; twenty incidents per year for two or more years was not uncommon.

Hepatitis: high incidence of known hepatitis or positive antigen tests; 10 percent had chronic hepatitis of five years or longer duration.

Non-specific urethritis: multiple presentations, sometimes chronic in that an individual will report 6 or 7 episodes per year for up to 8 years; higher doses and longer duration of antibiotics as condition became resistant to chemical intervention.

Dermatological eruptions: specific, palliative, and prophylactic use of antibiotics, tetracycline, and corticosteroids for skin eruptions; reports of prescribed tetracycline for 5 to 18 years continuously.

Sedatives, tranquilizers, and mood drugs: for psychological conditions; prescribed or used without prescription.

Chronic sore throat: more than 50 percent report frequent episodes [requiring] antibiotic medications.

Herpes simplex: 25 percent report chronic herpes; 90 percent herpes within the past 10 years.

Allergies: high incidence of history of chronic and severe allergies, allergy medications, and symptomatic suppressants.

Lymphadenopathy: frequent to chronic swollen lymph glands in 40 percent of sample for up to 25 years preceding survey.

Diarrhoea: high incidence of known and unknown etiologies; frequent parasites suspected, and parasitic treatments with and without confirmation of actual organisms in nearly 30 percent of our study.

Recreational drugs: nearly universal use of marijuana; a multiple and complex use of LSD, MDA, PCP, heroin, cocaine, amyl and butyl nitrites, amphetamines, barbiturates, ethyl chloride, opium, mush-rooms, and what are referred to as "designer drugs."[11]

One fourth of the sample shared nine or more of these con-ditions and patterns, and all individuals diagnosed as having AIDS or the AIDS-related complex (ARC) were concentrated in this smaller group.

Since this description probably characterizes a large por-tion of those who pursue the gay lifestyle, it can be seen that this lifestyle involves very heavy consumption of medications.

And, as we will show, all of these medications add a fur-ther burden of immunosuppression to the systems of those who may already suffer from syphilis or some other venereal disease.

Physicians give little thought to the possible immunosup-pressive effects of the medications they prescribe. Roger Finch, of the Nottingham City Hospital in England, wrote in 1980:

> The action of antimicrobial agents on the immune system is largely ignored in clinical practice, although a variety of effects — mostly in experimental systems — on both cell-mediated and humoral immunity have been recognized. . . . Among the many antimicrobial agents that have been studied, rifampicin, the tetra-cyclines, and the cephalosporins have attracted most attention.[12]

He observes further, "The relevance of many of these obser-vations is probably minor, since antimicrobial chemotherapy is usually short-lived . . . " That may be true for the popula-tion at large — but is less so for individuals in whom twenty "incidents" of gonorrhoea per year for two or more years are a fact of life.

The homosexual population, in particular, consumes these drugs regularly, *often on a prophylactic basis,* and thus suffers their full immunosuppressive effect.

What is the reaction of the potential AIDS patient, for example, to one of that year's 20 incidents of gonorrhoea? He will first seek an antimicrobial substance to rid himself of the gonococcus, and here one of the drugs of choice is tetracycline. In fact, tetracycline, as we will see, emerges as the preeminent prescribable for virtually every venereal disease, being used in the treatment not only of gonorrhoea and syphilis, but also lymphadenitis, non-venereal urethritis, pelvic inflammatory disease, vaginitis, vulvitis, lymph node enlargement, and other venereal diseases as well.

Its immunosuppressive effects have already been documented by us.

Among the common effects of chronic gonorrhoea are symptoms of gout and arthritis. The *National Disease and Therapeutic Index,* a quarterly trade publication of the pharmaceutical industry listing the medicines most commonly prescribed and the diseases for which they are given, notes "gout specifics" as the class of drugs most often given for gonorrhoea. And the leading "gout specific"—colchicine (*Col-BENEMID, Colprobenecid,* etc.)—acts directly on the bone marrow, impairing the production of white-blood cells ("leukopenia") and granulocytes ("agranulocytosis"), and sometimes causes aplastic anemia.

But this is not the end of the story.

The physician may prescribe one of the cephalosporins (marketed under such names as *Mefoxin, Cefobid, Keflex, Ancef, Ceclor, Velosef, Cefotan, Duricef, Rocephin, Keflin, Ultracef,* etc.) which are structurally very similar to penicillin and have similar adverse effects on the immune system: bone-marrow depression leading to impaired lymphocyte response and reduced numbers of granulocytes ("granulocytopenia") and thrombocytes ("thrombocytopenia"), as well as such allergic reactions as urticaria, maculopapular rashes, breathing difficulties caused by sudden constriction of the bronchial tubes ("bronchospasm"), and anaphylactic shock. The cephalosporins are prescribed for: vaginitis, candida infections, acute gonorrhoea, lymphadenitis, anal fistula, pelvic inflammatory disease and other infections of the female genital tract, non-venereal urethritis, lymph-node enlargement, vulvitis, and others.

Another class of antimicrobials are the sulfonamides, including trimethoprim/sulfamethoxazole (*Bactrim*), sulfisoxazole (*Gantrisin*), and many others. A leading textbook of pharmacology observes:

> The untoward events that follow the administration of sulfonamides are numerous and varied. They may involve nearly every organ system . . . The overall incidence of reactions is about 5 percent. Certain of these interdict the subsequent use of any sulfonamide; included in this category are drug fever and reactions involving the blood, bone marrow, kidney, liver, skin, and peripheral nerves . . . Complete suppression of bone-marrow activity with profound anemia, granulocytopenia, and thrombocytopenia is an extremely rare phenomenon with sulfonamide therapy. It probably results from a direct [bone-marrow] toxic effect, and may be fatal.[13]

The sulfonamide drugs are used to treat pelvic inflammatory disease, anal fistula, venereal diseases, vulvitis, vaginitis, etc. For these last two conditions *Sultrin: Triple Sulfa Cream and Vaginal Tablets* (containing sulphathiazole, sulfacetamide, and sulfabenzamide) is very popular.

□ □ □ □ □

But the treatment of gonorrhoea, syphilis, non-gonococcal urethritis, herpes, cytomegalovirus and Epstein-Barr virus infections, chlamydia and candida, and the whole host of venereal diseases that have arisen in the wake of the sexual revolution of recent decades involves many additional immunosuppressant drugs.

Skin rashes are among the most common symptoms of these diseases. Thus "dermatological and other preparations" are the No. 1 class of remedies prescribed for the class, "venereal disease," in the *National Disease and Therapeutic Index*.

Of these preparations, tetracycline ointments (*Topicycline, Achromycin ointment*) are very much at the forefront.

The various corticosteroids are also dispensed wholesale by physicians, and, since they are even advertised to the public on television, being available without a prescription, are consumed in large quantities without benefit of any sort of diagnosis. They are known to curtail the numbers of B- and T-lymphocytes in the circulating blood (lymphopenia) besides depressing the immune response in several other ways.

For the same condition, or perhaps for one of the dermatological consequences of gonorrhoea or syphilis, the patient might be prescribed prednisone (*Deltasone, Meticorten, Orasone, Sterapred,* etc.) which is so immunosuppressant that it is used to control the immune response and prevent rejection in organ transplant and skin graft operations.

Chloramphenicol (*Chloromycetin*), the first synthetic antibiotic, was one of the most frequently prescribed drugs in the pharmacopoeia until it was found to be highly toxic to bone marrow formation. It caused death from "blood dyscrasia," but, despite this history, is today being prescribed for "susceptible organisms which have been demonstrated to be resistant to all other appropriate antimicrobial agents" or "superficial skin infections caused by bacteria susceptible to chloramphenicol." One chloromycetin preparation, *Ophthochlor,* is used in the treatment of herpes-related ophthalmia. Another compound, *Ophthocort,* also used for ophthalmias, is contrived from cortisone and chloramphenicol and thus confers a dual immunosuppressive effect.

A chronic subclinical meningitis (meningismus) is sometimes associated with syphilis, and thus could also be open to treatment with chloramphenicol. Or a syphilis patient suspected of being a carrier of the meningitis microorganism

(*Neisseria meningitidis*) could be given rifampin (*Rifadin*), a classic bone-marrow depressant which also has a number of allergic effects.

Candida (moniliasis) and other fungal infections are extremely common in the population with venereal disease, leading to the use of such anti-fungal preparations as amphotericin-b (*Mysteclin*), clotrimazole (*Mycalex, Lotrimin, Lotrisone, Gyne-Lotrimin*), miconazole (*Monistat, Monistat-Derm*), and metronizadole (*Flagyl*). *Mysteclin* is often taken for ameba infections arising through physical contact with feces during rectal intercourse. *Mycalex* is used as a dermatologic cream or vaginal suppository against pruritus due to candida and other fungal overgrowths. *Flagyl* is probably the most frequently prescribed medication for vaginal itching.

In general, "vaginitis" and "vulvitis," meaning inflammation and itching in these regions, are treated with the whole panoply of immunosuppressants mentioned above: terramycin, vaginal sulfa drugs, cortisone creams, ampicillin, mycalex, doxycycline, cephalosporin, amoxycillin, erythromycin, and the like.

All of them have an adverse impact on the formation of lymphocytes and other components of the blood which participate in the organism's system of immune protection.

The female patient whose venereal disease has progressed to chronic pelvic infection—endometritis, nongonococcal tuboovarian abscess, pelvic cellulitis, or some similar condition—and who is allergic to penicillin, might get clindamycin (*Cleocin*) which is also known to impair bone-marrow synthesis of lymphocytes and other components of the blood.

Ironically, these medicines can in some cases cause the very conditions for which they are prescribed. The product insert for *Mysteclin* observes:

> Candidal overgrowth occurs in a large number of patients taking broad-spectrum antibiotics. Although it is impossible to predict exactly which patient will

develop candidal complications and which will not, certain types of patients are known to be particularly susceptible to candidiasis. Among these are elderly or debilitated patients, patients on high or prolonged antibiotic dosage; diabetics; infants [?]; patients on corticoid therapy; patients who have developed candidiasis on previous broad-spectrum therapy; women [?], particularly during pregnancy . . . indicated for the many common infections, including those of the respiratory, gastrointestinal, and genitourinary systems, which are amenable to tetracycline therapy. Infections caused by gram-positive and gram-negative bacteria, spirochetes [!] . . . and Endamoeba histolytica can be expected to respond. Because of the wide range of antimicrobial activity, the preparations are particularly useful in the treatment of mixed infections due to susceptible organisms.[14]

How often has the medicine given for candida actually served to intensify the infestation, provoking the prescription of ever-larger doses, and so on, ad infinitum?

By the same token, allergy to ampicillin—used in the treatment of gonorrhoea and syphilis—has been diagnosed as secondary syphilis; the rash was found in one study to occur in almost 5 percent of patients. This is merely one more of many already confusing factors in the diagnosis and treatment of syphilis.[15]

The above are only a sampling of some of the more prominent agents involved in immunosuppression. We have stressed the medicines which act adversely on the bone marrow and its production of blood components, since this aspect of immunity is significantly related both to syphilis and to AIDS. We have also discussed the potential for causing hypersensitivity reactions. But there are other mechanisms of immune protection, and little is known about how they are affected by these and other medications.

The immune system is a highly complex system of defense which is by no means entirely understood by medicine today. Its principal characteristic is resourcefulness. An authority writes: "What I wish to emphasize at the outset is the singular flexibility of response made possible by the complex organization of the cellular and molecular components of the immune system. In almost no instance is the organism limited to one possible pathway in response to a . . . stimulus."[16] The immune response involves every aspect of the body's functioning, since any mechanism can be called into action when needed for purposes of protection. Thus interference by a drug with any aspect of the body's functioning can have reverberations on its system of immune response.

ロ ロ ロ ロ ロ

The typical AIDS patient is also likely to be a consumer of illegal drugs. The immunosuppressant action of these so-called "street" or "recreational" drugs should not be underrated. Marijuana, for instance, can induce immunologic deficiencies in the test-tube and perhaps in humans. Cocaine has been associated epidemiologically with KS and also with alterations in T-lymphocyte patterns in the blood. And, as already mentioned, amyl and butyl nitrite "poppers" used as "room odorizers," sexual stimulants, and anal muscle relaxants have also been associated with abnormal T-lymphocyte patterns.

These may well be major co-factors in the production of AIDS, but they should not deflect attention from therapeutic drugs whose immunosuppressive impact, all in all, is probably far greater.

Of course, the patient with AIDS and its associated infections will often be treated with these same, and other, immunosuppressant drugs. One authority recommends "early aggressive antimicrobial therapy" and even "long-term prophylaxis" with such drugs as trimethoprim/sulfamethoxazole ("the treatment of choice for PCP"), pentamidine (*Pentam*—"immediate toxicity is observed in many patients, manifesting

as hypotension, tachycardia, and facial flushing . . . Renal toxicity, hepatotoxicity, or both usually are reversible, but have
been reported in about 25 percent of patients receiving pentamidine"), vidaribine (*Vira-A* — "central nervous system distur-
bances have been reported at therapeutic doses . . . Hemato-
logic clinical laboratory changes noted . . . were a decrease in
hemoglobin or hematocrit, white blood cell count, and platelet
count . . ."), cytaribine (a "potent bone-marrow suppressant"
used also in cancer chemotherapy), acyclovir (*Zovirax*) for
herpes infections:

> Among 51 immunocompromised patients, one, a bone
> marrow transplant recipient with pneumonitis, de-
> veloped seizures, cerebral edema, coma, and expired
> with changes consistent with cerebral anoxia on post-
> mortem biopsy . . . Less frequent adverse reactions
> were . . . jitters [!]

as well as our old friends, amphotericin B, rifadin, corticosteroids, and others equally immunosuppressive.[17]

The warning given by Joseph Sonnabend in 1983, "Treatment of patients with AIDS with potent immunosuppressive
drugs may be very deleterious,"[18] seems to have gone un-
heeded.

□ □ □ □ □

Africans and Haitians are perhaps exposed to even greater
pharmacological risks than Americans and West Europeans.
In these countries antibiotics and other imported medicines
have long been seen as possessing particularly powerful magic.
They are much more easily available without prescription than
in the developed countries and are even sold on street cor-
ners. African hospital workers steal them from the dispen-
saries, then dilute them and sell them at retail to their friends
and acquaintances. Physicians in Zimbabwe wrote in 1985:
"Substantially more antibiotics are dispensed in Zimbabwe

compared to the U.K. and the U.S.A., with penicillins being used most frequently. Sulphonamides and tetracyclines were the next most frequently dispensed groups respectively."[19] Two other physicians reported in the same year: "The widespread usage of antibiotics in primary health care facilities without reference to laboratory evidence of its need is a cause for real concern and may be an important factor in the development and spread of resistant strains of potential pathogens . . . In developing countries misuse or overuse of common antibiotics obtained from a variety of sources may be an important factor in the emergence of drug resistance. Where financial resources are limited, great reliance is made on a limited range of relatively inexpensive antibiotics, and the development of resistance to these may therefore be a serious health problem."[20] Patients also prefer injections to orally administered medicines, which only exacerbates the situation.[21]

□ □ □ □ □

The possibility of immune-system suppression by drug therapy has, like the possibility of suppression through venereal disease, not been altogether ignored in the literature, but it is not given sufficient emphasis.

A 1985 article by staff of the Centers for Disease Control observes that "whether other factors that suppress the immune system, such as medical use of steroids . . . [or] other coexisting immunosuppressant diseases . . . may increase the risk of AIDS in persons infected with [AIDS virus] is unknown." But, after finding AIDS in some developing countries to be associated with "the number of injections received for therapeutic and nontherapeutic purposes," the authors blame "reuse of nonsterile needles"[22] and ignore the possibility that therapeutic injections themselves might be at fault. Lawrence Altman, medical journalist for the *New York Times,* notes without comment the theory that the AIDS virus "could have mutated in some unknown way as a reaction to the widespread use of antibiotics."[23]

This is not a popular line to pursue, however. The "cure" of syphilis with antibiotics was one of the medical triumphs of the 1950's; recognition of a reservoir of uncured syphilis in the treated population would raise a host of unanswered questions about the overuse of penicillin and other antibiotics in recent decades. Since these drugs are the foundation of modern therapeutics, no one is anxious to put such issues on the agenda. And yet they must be put on the agenda. The continuing assault on the immune system from the drugs used in modern medicine has helped prepare the ground for the modern scourge of AIDS.

6

The AIDS Virus
a Co-Factor?

The previous chapters have shown that it was an error to overlook preexisting syphilis and antibiotic abuse as factors making for vulnerability and facilitating the spread of the AIDS virus. The condition of the victim, the "host organism," should be at the center of attention.

But nearly all discussion of AIDS has focussed on one or another supposed causal virus and ignored the victim. This was a mistake. All other diseases involve interaction between the causal organism and the host. Why should AIDS be an exception?

And this mistake is all the more inexcusable in light of the controversy over whether or not the AIDS virus really is *the* causal factor, or even *a* causal factor.

Some authorities would exonerate this virus altogether. A recent analysis by professor of molecular biology Peter Duesberg of the University of California, Berkeley, concludes that "AIDS virus is not sufficient to cause AIDS and . . . there is no evidence, besides its presence in a latent form, that it is necessary for AIDS . . . AIDS virus could be just the most common occupational infection of those at risk for AIDS."[1]

His judgment is supported by accounts of nurses and other health workers inadvertently injecting themselves with AIDS-contaminated blood — the so-called "needlestick infections" — without any harmful consequences. A typical case was reported in 1984: a nurse in England jabbed her finger while resheathing a hypodermic needle used on an AIDS patient and probably injected herself with the patient's blood; thirteen days later she came down with a severe influenza-like illness, followed by sore throat, headache, muscle aches, facial neuralgia, and then a non-itching macular rash; she also had arthritic pains and general lymphadenopathy but recovered spontaneously in three or four weeks without taking any medication.[2] In 1985 a nurse in France pricked her finger with a needle used to take blood from an AIDS patient; two months later she had a fever and a macular eruption which progressively covered her face, arms, and thorax; the illness resolved in three days, and blood tests showed that she had antibodies to the AIDS virus; a year later she was in good health.[3] Major Robert Redfield, who is one of the U.S. Army's chief AIDS researchers, twice stuck himself with needles full of virus-loaded cells and one of those times injected a large number of cells into his arm; he did not even fall sick.[4]

A 1985 review article found that by April, 1984, there had been 31 such accidents, involving 30 persons. The authors reported: "These subjects have remained healthy"; none had even developed antibodies against the virus.[5] Later that same year the total had risen to 40, but all were healthy, and none had developed antibodies over a median follow-up period of 8.5 months.[6] By March 31, 1987 over 1224 needlestick cases had been reported to the Centers for Disease Control. Of these only 370 cases had been comprehensively tested, but it appeared that only one person had even developed AIDS-virus antibodies, while none had become sick with AIDS or even with the AIDS-related syndrome (ARC).[7]

These figures suggest that truly healthy persons will not become sick with AIDS, or die from it, merely through exposure to the virus, while only three exposed persons in 1000 will even develop antibodies.

It might be objected that AIDS is known to develop slowly and that persons like the above who have been strongly exposed to the AIDS virus will eventually fall ill with the disease. Perhaps a year or so is too short a follow-up period.

However, there is evidence against this also. Surveys in a number of third-world countries have documented very wide dissemination of the AIDS virus in these countries while the bearers of the virus lead healthy and uneventful lives. Investigators are forced to conclude that people may have been living for a generation or more with this virus, which causes them no particular harm.

For instance, in a remote rural area of Eastern Zaire 250 patients from a local hospital, none of whom had clinical AIDS, were tested in 1985; 12 percent showed a clear presence of AIDS-virus antibodies, while another 12 percent were borderline. The incidence was highest among uneducated agricultural workers, and the authors concluded that the virus, or one closely related to it, was endemic in the region. "Among the subjects with antibodies in this survey there was no correlation with any symptoms of illness or acute or non-acute health complaints, suggesting that these subjects were not ill with any of the AIDS-related health problems described in current epidemics . . . Thus, if antibodies indicate prior exposure to [the AIDS virus], this population must have had and survived [AIDS-virus] infection without lasting health problems."[8] In 1985 Venezuelan Indians who live in complete isolation from the rest of the country's population were found to manifest an incidence of 3.3 to 13.3 percent infection with the AIDS virus; being out of contact with modern civilization, these Indians were extremely unlikely to have been recently infected.[9]

These facts cast very serious doubt on the lethality of the AIDS virus in the absence of a notable cofactor. In our view, a history of syphilis is the indispensable cofactor.

While Duesberg would eliminate the AIDS virus from consideration, others are proposing different candidates.

One is the "African green monkey virus," which is a near cousin of the AIDS virus. The green monkey is an important article of diet in some parts of Africa; the virus is thought to have entered the food chain and in this way become a cause of AIDS. Scientists are perplexed, however, by the fact that the green monkey virus is perfectly innocuous; why the almost identical AIDS virus should be so threatening is a puzzle.[10]

An even more promising candidate is the virus of African Swine Fever (ASF) which may also have become infectious to man via the food chain. In 1983 Jane Teas, of the Harvard School of Public Health, was the first to call attention to a possible link between the 1978 appearance of AIDS in Haiti and the 1979 epidemic of African Swine Fever on that island. It was already known that many Haitians had been living in Zaire in the 1960's when they were brought in to do the work of the departing Belgian administrators; when they returned to Haiti, they could have brought the swine fever virus back with them. The Haitian farmers were encouraged to kill and eat infected pigs and could have picked up the virus in this way. There are many symptomatic and pathological parallels between AIDS and this disease — fever, swelling of the lymph nodes, skin and brain lesions, and pneumonia. Later it could have passed to the United States through contact with homosexual tourists for whom Haiti was once a favored vacation spot.[11]

Throughout 1986 Teas and her associate, John Beldekas, feuded with the U.S. Department of Agriculture and the Centers for Disease Control over the validity of this causal hypothesis. Teas and Beldekas claimed to have found: (1) evidence of the ASF virus in the swine population of Belle Glade, Florida, a town of 15,000 poor agricultural workers, including many Haitian immigrants, on the shores of Lake Okeechobee which is known as the "AIDS capital of the U.S." for the large number of AIDS cases found there; (2) evidence of infection of these same hogs with the AIDS virus; (3) evidence of infection of American AIDS patients with the ASF virus.[12]

With both the AIDS virus and the ASF virus found in both pigs and AIDS patients, there seemed to be at least a plausible hypothesis for investigation. Moreover, the New York City Health Department had already announced in September, 1985, that a random test of 160 blood donors at the New York Blood Center disclosed that 5 showed evidence of infection with the ASF.[13] One of these five, additionally, showed evidence of infection with the AIDS virus itself. ASF infection had never before been documented in humans.[14]

At this point, however, Teas and Beldekas found themselves blocked. When they first produced their data on ASF virus in the Belle Glade hogs, the USDA admitted that at least one pig had tested positive for antibody to the ASF virus. Later, however, the USDA and the CDC retested the Belle Glade swine and a group of AIDS patients and concluded that the earlier finding was a mistake.[15] "We found no evidence of ASFV infection in people with [AIDS] infection or of [AIDS] infection in pigs."[16]

The New York City Health Department data have also dropped through the cracks. The Health Commissioner announced, "This [sic] preliminary screening data do not support the hypothesis of an association between [the AIDS virus] and African Swine Fever Virus." But that was hardly the question. The data were far too sketchy to support, or to disprove, the hypothesis. But they should have aroused curiosity. As Jane Teas has commented, "They should have been asking themselves how the African Swine Fever Virus, which is supposedly unknown in the United States, could show up in 5 out of 160 random blood samples in New York City. At the least, this should have led to further investigations and further sampling." In fact, no one has pursued this matter further, and the CDC itself never even commented on the data of the New York City Health Department.

The whole question has become entangled in a mass of

charges and countercharges, of contradictory test results, and of assertions that the ASF virus is cross-reacting with other viruses and thus skewing test results.[17]

African Swine Fever is a very serious illness. When it first appeared among European swine imported into Kenya in 1910, the mortality was close to 100 percent. Today it is much lower, but the illness leaves the pigs debilitated and subject to other sicknesses. Furthermore, ASF-virus-contaminated pork could not be exported from the United States. Possibly for this reason the USDA has refused to allow Teas and Beldekas to use its facility on Plum Island (Long Island Sound) to test their hypothesis. A spokesman stated: "If the virus got out, it could devastate the pork industry." But the USDA seems to fear that even talk of a possible connection with the African Swine Fever might have a devastating impact on pork exports.

Every aspect of the AIDS issue has been entangled in politics from the very outset. The category "Haitian" was eliminated from the statistics of incidence. The U.S. pork industry objects to discussing the African Swine Fever. And the possibility that AIDS is related to underlying syphilis and the abuse of antibiotics has not been mentioned at all. These examples show that supposedly scientific or medical issues have enormous political, social, and economic dimensions which may have a decisive influence on how the purely medical aspects are discussed and resolved.

But AIDS is a qualitatively new challenge. This sort of "politics as usual" may no longer be good enough as the death rate continues to rise.

☐ ☐ ☐ ☐ ☐

AIDS can probably be caused by a number of different microorganisms in an immunosuppressed host. Various scenarios can be imagined. Precisely which virus could be the cause is an interesting topic for research, but probably less important for treatment, which should focus on the devastated immune systems of the potential AIDS victims. Today they are sitting ducks for whatever virus happens to be playing the role of cofactor.

This point has been made by others. Researchers from the National Cancer Institute and the Danish Institute of Cancer Research observed in 1985 that the different incidence of AIDS in the various risk groups "may reflect duration of exposure in a cohort but also factors such as source, route, and dose of exposure, *environmental factors such as infections or immune-altering exposure* [stress added] . . ."[18] Two associates of the Cancer Research Institute of the University of California School of Medicine in San Francisco wrote in 1983 that "AIDS is itself an opportunistic infection. It causes disease only in individuals who are already immunocompromised by hepatitis-B, cytomegalovirus, parasites, or other immunosuppressive factors . . . immunologically competent individuals are not at risk of acquiring the syndrome . . ."[19] Peter Duesberg concludes that "the disease would then be caused by an as yet unidentified agent which may not even be a virus . . . However, the virus may be responsible for the early, mononucleosis-like disease observed in several infections . . ."[20]

This realization should serve to supply some perspective on AIDS and make us wary of statements like the one made by Robert Gallo, that "normal healthy people with no disease symptoms at all who aren't sexually active, who are not IV-drug users" are not free of risk.[21] It seems unlikely that the completely healthy and syphilis-free person whose immune system functions properly would contract anything worse than a more or less severe mononucleosis if exposed to the AIDS virus, like the health workers who stick their fingers with infected hypodermic needles.

The great majority — who do not have 1000 sexual partners per year, who have never had syphilis, and who do not consume "street" or "medicinal" drugs on a regular basis — are probably risk-free, even if the AIDS virus, or antibodies to it, can be found in the bloodstream. Jacques Leibowitch's recent book, *A Strange Virus of Unknown Origin*, states that "possibly less than ten percent of those carrying the virus will ever experience any symptoms at all."[22]

A substantial part of the population in most countries of the world tests positive for tuberculosis, indicating previous infection. The disease, however, occurs only in those whose health is impaired for other reasons.

The presence of AIDS virus in the tissues of a healthy individual should cause concern only when associated with the presence, or the threat, of syphilis.

7

Prevention
and Treatment

AIDS is not just a disease like other diseases. It is to some extent a man-made catastrophe and must be classified with other destructive environmental effects of man's activities.

This time, however, it is our internal environment which is being assaulted and destroyed.

AIDS is the long-term price paid for a short-term benefit and is thus the medical parallel of our depletion of the ozone layer, the destruction of tropical rain forests, the burdening of the atmosphere with sulphuric acid from coal-fired power installations, the poisoning of rivers and oceans with pesticides.

The short-term benefit has been the quick cure of illnesses with antibiotics. The long-term price is impairment of the immune system.

Enough has been written elsewhere about the baneful impact of certain types of sexual activities, especially among homosexuals. Obviously multiple anonymous sexual liaisons are debilitating in a variety of ways. Obviously repeated infection with secondary venereal diseases, in addition to continuous intimate oral and anal contact with semen and feces, is, on the whole, bad for the health. That this should progressively undermine the immune system is not in any way astonishing.

But due notice has not yet been taken of the great ancestral venereal disease which has shadowed the human race since the fifteenth century and which is still only partially understood. Maltreatment of the post-war syphilis epidemic drove this scourge underground, preparing its victims for infestation with a new set of viruses.

Thus one major cause of AIDS is the progressive disabling of millions of immune systems by uncured syphilis. The other major cause is found in the very drugs which have been used to treat this syphilis (and most other diseases besides). Modern "scientific" medical practice relies very largely on medicines whose ultimate effect is to impair the patient's immune system.

This is no secret, no great discovery. It is discussed in all the relevant literature. But it has never seemed significant until today when the world is faced with an epidemic rooted in a pervasive crippling of the immune system. The drugs synthesized since the end of World War II have achieved their end — the antibiotic sterilization, more or less, of patients' bodies — at the expense of the immune system, and AIDS is the last stop on the line. The immune system cannot be suppressed and undermined indefinitely without a price being paid. The chickens have come home to roost.

□ □ □ □ □

What does all this signify for prevention and cure?

Clearly prevention is more promising than treatment. The danger of AIDS can be warded off by avoiding actions and substances which damage the immune system. This includes exaggerated sexual practices and exaggerated consumption of therapeutic or non-therapeutic drugs. Anyone with an ongoing syphilis infection will have to take particular care to avoid concomitant exposure to the AIDS virus.

The treatment of AIDS is very much on the agenda. It

undoubtedly offers less promising prospects than prevention of the disease, but here also some possibilities exist.

If our causal analysis is correct, AIDS will not be successfully treated by a drug which inhibits or annihilates the virus. No therapy directed at the "causal" virus, rather than the immune-compromised host, will be promising. Thus a medication such as AZT (axidothymidine) will never do patients any good, however expensive it may be and whatever scientific "breakthroughs" it may represent. It will only distract them from more promising modes of treatment.

On the other hand, if AIDS is generated by an underlying syphilis, its treatment by high doses of penicillin might offer hope. And if positive results are attained, this would perhaps be proof of the syphilis connection.

One physician who has pursued this hypothesis is Stephen Caiazza, of New York City, who has been mentioned earlier (see Appendix B). After treating AIDS patients for several years with various recommended drugs and seeing all of them die, he discovered that many had been infected with syphilis. This led him to test his other patients, and he found that, when the FTA and more sophisticated tests were used, nearly all turned out to be positive for syphilis. "We suspect," he states, "that AIDS is caused primarily by virulent immunosuppressive treponemes with the AIDS virus functioning in a manner still undefined, but presumably as a permissive and/or synergistic cofactor. The so-called 'AIDS virus' masks the presence of syphilis and confounds our ability to detect it."

By now Caiazza and his associates have treated several dozen patients on the syphilis hypothesis. They recommend intravenous aqueous penicillin (40 million units a day for twenty days) for its ability to penetrate the blood-brain barrier, but since this must be given intravenously in a hospital setting, for out-patients they prescribe oral doxycycline, which also penetrates the blood-brain barrier, as well as benzathine penicillin and oral tetracycline, depending on the patient's condition and circumstances.

This treatment is essentially the same as aggressive treatment for tertiary syphilis. As such, it threatens further immune-system suppression, but patients who are desperate are willing to run this risk. While Caiazza has been following this program for only a short time, he claims that some patients already show signs of improvement — feeling better, putting on weight, and resuming a normal life.

It is still too early to judge whether the penicillin treatment is fully successful, but if Caiazza's patients do not relapse, it will be strong evidence in favor of the syphilis hypothesis.

As Caiazza observes, because penicillin is inexpensive and unprotected by patent, some elements in the medical-industrial complex will oppose its use. In these circles there is always an animus in favor of expensive modes of treatment over inexpensive ones (AZT, for instance, is estimated to cost each patient $10,000 per year while promising nothing more than marginal postponement of the moment of death).[1] This factor should be borne in mind in future debates over treatment.*

But the penicillin treatment of AIDS is fighting fire with fire and cannot go on indefinitely.

Alternatives must be sought, and one which has been under active investigation involves measures to strengthen the immune system. Some work is already being done on transfusing lymphocytes, replacing bone marrow, transplanting thymic tissue, and the like. Medications are also being sought which in principle stimulate the immune system. Alpha and gamma interferon, Interleukin-2, inosine pranobex (*Isoprinosine*), azimexon, cimetidine and others have all been tried,

---

*Needless to say, the stampede to bring other untested medicines to the market, without first undergoing scrutiny by the FDA, should be resisted to the utmost. Relaxation of regulatory control will merely open the doors wide to any substance that can be synthesized rapidly by an enterprising manufacturer armed with a plausible etiological theory of AIDS.

but no perceptible clinical results have yet been achieved. What Anthony Fauci and H. Clifford Lane stated in 1985 is still true today: "At present, no effective therapy is available for the underlying immune defect seen in patients with AIDS."[2]

Unfortunately, a whole body of scientific information on strengthening the immune system has been entirely ignored. This is homoeopathic medicine, which employs small doses of a variety of therapeutic drugs to challenge the immune system and provoke a response. Thus it seems peculiarly well suited to the treatment of AIDS.[3]

Indeed, because it has always been oriented toward the recuperative potential of the patient's immune system rather than toward annihilating the microbial "causes" of diseases, homoeopathy has consistently been characterized as "unscientific" by the dominant school of medical thought. Perhaps the time has now come to revise that opinion.

Naturopathic medicine, which is a group of therapeutic procedures including homoeopathy, also offers promise in the treatment of AIDS.

Furthermore, homoeopathic and naturopathic practitioners find that the most commonly indicated homoeopathic medicines are ones traditionally employed in the treatment of syphilis. Such remedies as *Mercurius, Arsenicum album, Sulphur,* and *Nitric acid* which are well-known homoeopathic standbys for treating this venereal disease crop up very frequently in the differential diagnosis and therapeutics of AIDS.[4]

This is one more piece of evidence in favor of the identity of AIDS and syphilis.

Maurice Jenaer, M.D., of Brussels, treats AIDS patients in Belgium and also in Zaire with homoeopathic preparations of DNA, RNA, and cyclosporin (which was for a while extolled as a general treatment for AIDS by orthodox medicine).[5]

The naturopathic school, which is particularly strong in the states of Oregon and Washington, has many other techniques for treating AIDS in addition to the classic homoeopathic syphilis remedies. The clinic of the National College of Naturopathic Medicine, in Portland, Oregon, administers from 12 to 60 grams of vitamin C per day to its patients, as well as other vitamins, herbal remedies, and minerals, and compels the patients to follow a strict dietary regimen involving abstention from sugar, alcohol, nicotine, drugs, and processed foods.[6] Joan McKenna and her associates in Berkeley, California, have a similar program.

Much information on the homoeopathic and naturopathic treatment of AIDS has been incorporated in the book, *Healing AIDS Naturally*, by Laurence Badgley, M.D. As the title suggests, the book seeks to cure AIDS by supporting the body's own natural powers of recuperation or, in other words, by stimulating the immune system.[7]

These unorthodox procedures have always stressed a therapeutic approach which builds up the patient's own powers of immune resistance. While this approach has been derided in the past by those who thought that only their medicine was "scientific," the time is now at hand when this skill will be increasingly in demand.

□ □ □ □ □

To conclude, there is a little good news mixed with a lot of bad.

In the first place, AIDS is unlikely to spread like wildfire to completely healthy persons. While predictions are always risky, the Sodom and Gomorrah scenario of destruction visited on a quarter of the earth's population seems wildly exaggerated. In fact, the disease is unlikely to spread beyond the existing reservoir of persons whose immune systems are in a shambles due a combination of endemic syphilis and intensive use of immunosuppressive medication.

The bad news is that the number of cases continues to rise. Indeed, the reservoir of potential candidates is large. Syphilis has been endemic for centuries in many parts of the world, and modern medical practice relies almost exclusively on medicines with a pronouncedly immunosuppressive effect.* Anyone with these two predisposing factors in his background is vulnerable to infection with one or another of the viruses which can lead to AIDS.

What is worse, these viruses are becoming endemic and may now represent a permanent threat to the health of anyone with an impaired immune system. They are a sword of Damocles hanging over all who pursue a lifestyle which damages and impairs the immune system, whether this involves multiple homosexual or heterosexual relationships, long-term use of "street drugs" or systematic use of therapeutic ones.

□ □ □ □ □

The AIDS epidemic also conveys a notable message to physicians. If their ever-expanding use of immunosuppressive drugs is contributing to the pool of individuals at risk to contract AIDS, they must revise therapeutic practice, and, indeed, therapeutic theory, to encourage less destructive modes of treatment.

But the use of these violent medications is supported and bolstered by a whole theoretical construct known as "scientific medicine," and many M.D.'s will feel that warding off the challenge of AIDS means abjuring "scientific medicine."

However, a system of medicine whose long-term effect is to impair the patient's immune system can hardly be a reputable "science."

Science is only a way of harnessing the forces of nature to attain a desired end. Destruction of the immune system cannot be such a desired aim of medicine; ergo, the "science" which brings this about should be replaced by a different

---

*Indeed, the whole lifestyle of modern industrial society, with its various environmental contaminants, sources of radiation, food additives, and the like, undermines and breaks down the immune system.

science.

There is more than one way to elaborate a medical science, and the alternatives should be investigated.

Even the fact that physicians must once again come to grips with the perennial problem of syphilis will compel a certain revision and reconstruction of medical ideas. This disease was thought to have been conquered and eliminated, and now it is visiting us once again. What went wrong in the past?

If AIDS really is an "iatrogenic disease"—i.e., caused, at least in part, by physicians—the procedures generating it should be revised. If it really is the price being paid for past "successes," these "successes" should be reevaluated.

The medical profession should stop fantasizing about (God help us!) vaccinating the whole population and examine more closely the homegrown causes of the AIDS scourge.[8]

It should seek a different theory and practice of drug treatment, to avoid the immuno-destructive consequences of those presently in use.

It should verify the extent to which syphilis and antibiotic medicines are causal agents of this condition by inquiring, far more pertinaciously than is done at present, into the venereal disease background of all those with AIDS or the AIDS-related complex, and their consumption of therapeutic drugs.

These steps should be taken immediately. Delay merely expands the pool of potential victims.

□ □ □ □ □

Finally, we should be aware that AIDS research and practice—like all other areas of medical activity—involves psychological, political, and economic motivations as well as scientific. These may well be unconscious, with the physicians and scientists involved being unaware of the extent to which their thinking is guided by them. We maintain that the sudden and unexpected onslaught of AIDS has to some extent panicked the American medical establishment, causing it to overlook the syphilis connection which otherwise should be quite evi-

cent. Their psychological vulnerability is supported by a series of political and economic factors which make it essential that AIDS be interpreted as a wholly new phenomenon and not the resurgence of a well-known disease from the past. The interviews with Joan McKenna and Stephen Caiazza (Appendices A and B) describe in graphic detail what are the psychological, political, and economic barriers to a new theory of AIDS today.

But these barriers cannot remain in place forever. The increasing numbers of AIDS patients will insist on a trial of penicillin, and the public will refuse to continue financing an increasingly expensive program of research and treatment based on a wrong theory of the disease's origins.

Appendix A

Interview with
Joan McKenna

Joan McKenna, of the Institute for Thermobaric Studies, Berkeley, California, was the first person in the United States to systematically investigate the connection between AIDS and syphilis. This interview was recorded in June, 1987.

HLC: Let me start by asking what has been the reaction to your pioneering article on AIDS and syphilis which appeared last December in *Medical Hypotheses.**

JMcK: The best reaction was a January 16, 1987, editorial in the AMA *Journal* by Mary E. Guinan of the CDC which pointed out that serological tests are not a real criterion of cure in syphilis, that the penicillin treatment of syphilis is still controversial, and that if the individual is immune-suppressed from prior disease — such as AIDS — or drugs or anything else,

---

*J. J. McKenna *et al.*, "Unmasking AIDS: Chemical Immunosuppression and Seronegative Syphilis." *Medical Hypotheses* 21:4 (December, 1986), 421–430.

the penicillin could be ineffective.* Thus the CDC seems to be picking up on the points we made in our *Medical Hypotheses* article.

In the meantime, of course, we had been moving the information around. In the summer of 1986 I went to Europe and talked to specialists in London, at the Institute for Tropical Diseases, and at the World Health Organization in Geneva. I talked to Klaus-Uwe Dierig and Urban Waldthaler in Augsburg, West Germany. They had earlier published an article in a West German medical journal describing a history of syphilis in one AIDS patient and gonorrhoea in another AIDS patient. They suspected from this that AIDS was a deep-seated venereal disease, so they gave the patients 40 million units a day of penicillin-G for 20 days, and after 12–15 months they were free of symptoms.†

HLC: So you're saying that you and these West German physicians were working independently and in parallel on the AIDS/syphilis connection?

JMcK: Yes.

HLC: Tell me how you hit on this idea in the first place.

JMcK: It started about 6 years ago, in 1981. The reason was that I didn't believe what I was reading about AIDS in the newspapers. It wasn't consistent with what I knew about the gay community and about AIDS.

We've known for a long time that the gay community is subject to a lot of chronic inflammatory conditions. And that they use a lot of drugs which are immunosuppressive. And that these give rise to a "syndrome," a condition of the organism, which predisposes to such secondary infections as,

---

*Mary E. Guinan, "Treatment of Primary and Secondary Syphilis: Defining Failure at Three- and Six-Month Follow-up" (editorial). *JAMA* 257:3 (January16, 1987), 359–360.

†Klaus-Uwe Dierig and Urban Waldthaler, "Perspektive aus der Praxis: Immundefekt — ein Vorstadium?" *Selecta* 36 (September 9, 1985), 3231–3235.

for instance, *Pneumocystis carinii* pneumonia.

In England or Europe, when you have one of these secondary infections, the physician will say, "Tell me every drug you've taken in the last six months, and don't lie about it!!" And then he will ask you if you've had any of the following diseases and give you a whole list of chronic inflammatory diseases. Then he will ask about environmental exposure to radiation, various toxic chemicals, etc. From this he can usually figure out what is causing the syndrome.

You can't catch a syndrome after all. It's quite specific to the individual patient and to the set of circumstances or forces that change the total response of his system to the microorganisms that are indigenous to it.

What the CDC seemed to be doing was to change the rules. It was saying that the AIDS epidemic just arose out of nowhere, with no grounds for it. It was ignoring the factors which caused this syndrome. Specifically, it seemed to be saying that, in looking at the gay community, prostitutes, intravenous drug abusers, and the like, there were no previous chronic inflammatory diseases, while drug use played no role at all.

HLC: They were turning things upside down?

JMcK: Yes, for some reason they were denying that drugs were a major problem in these communities, and they were denying that physicians had anything to do with prescribed drugs being abused substances in these communities.

HLC: You can understand why they would deny that.

JMcK: Maybe so, but to say that these individuals didn't have chronic inflammatory conditions is really beyond me.

HLC: OK, so you started in 1981. What was the first thing you did?

JMcK: I started with a literature search on acquired immunodeficiency syndromes and documented the history of this. I found an account of a European epidemic of PCP in orphan asylums after World War II; it turned out that the children were getting antibiotics like penicillin and terramycin prophylactically. So the PCP was generated in their chemically altered immune systems.

One reason why in hospitals today they are so nervous about AIDS is that everyone being treated with anti-inflammatories for chronic inflammatory diseases, such as rheumatoid arthritis, or being given chemical immunosuppressives, essentially has a kind of pre-AIDS syndrome.

Anyway, to go back to our chronology, it struck me that from what I knew about the gay community, they had a history of chronic inflammatory disease and chronic drug abuse, and the first thing to do was to stop that. So in 1981 I started a program to help them — a program of life-style changes that would enable them to live without drugs and would remove some of the burden of their chronic inflammations.

HLC: When did you first catch on to the syphilis connection?

JMcK: About 1983. By this time my first AIDS patient had been three years without complications. His physician was referring people to me. Other people had heard about my program and wanted to get in. I couldn't handle so many clients on a one-to-one basis, so I set up a training module. We ended up working with about 100 people, 32 with AIDS and the rest with ARC (AIDS-related complex) or simply the "worried well."

What we were really trying to do was to help them get their immune systems back into shape. As it was, they simply didn't have any reactive ability. Once we managed to restore some life to their immune systems, however, we found a funny thing happening. All of a sudden they started developing fevers. This meant they were reacting, since a fever is a sign of the body's reaction. It is part of a curative process. But what were they reacting to?

Furthermore, these fevers seemed to have no other accompanying phenomena, no other symptoms, no distinctive biochemical findings. They were just cyclical spiking fevers apparently isolated from any pathological basis.

So I said this is crazy, I have to look into the literature to find out what is happening. About 1984 I was reading in the library of the UC Medical Center, San Francisco, and I came on an article that said point-blank, "Be careful not to confuse PCP with syphilis; both of them have a typical 'white lung' condition."* This really made me stop and think, "Could AIDS be a form of syphilis?"

And syphilis kept coming up again and again. I found a lot of articles from the 1950's and 1960's stating that you had to be very careful with subcurative penicillin treatment of syphilis, since the disease could skip the primary and secondary stages and go right into latency, and when it emerges later, it does so in very bizarre ways. I found more recent articles, such as the ones by Raymond Smego and Stephen McPhee stating that AIDS could easily be confused with secondary syphilis. † I found articles, beginning in the early 1950's, describing the successful treatment of KS with penicillin, i.e., with the drug which is used to treat syphilis.* † *

In 1984 I realized that suppression with medicinal drugs was one of the causes of AIDS and started talking about it. I am an optimist. I thought it was wonderful to understand the causes of things and be able to go to work on them. I didn't realize what was going on out there in the medical world that made it very hard for them to hear me. In a word, all hell broke loose, and I saw that this was an error on my part.

---

*Harald Gormsen, "On Interstitial Plasma Cell Pneumonia in Infants." *Acta Paediatrica* 39 (1950), 291–314.

†Raymond A. Smego *et al.*, "Secondary Syphilis Masquerading as AIDS in a Young Gay Male." *North Carolina Medical Journal* 45 (1984). 253–254. Stephen J. McPhee, "Secondary Syphilis: Uncommon Manifestations of a Common Disease." *Western Journal of Medicine* 140 (1984), 35.

*†*See the references in J. Fayolle *et al.*, "La Penicilline dans le Traitement de l'Angiosarcomatose de Kaposi: Rappel d'une thérapeutique oubliée à propos d'une observation." *Lyon Medical* 244:17 (1980), 277–281.

HLC: You mean that the doctors didn't want to be told that the drugs they were prescribing could suppress the patient's immune system and predispose him to AIDS?

JMcK: Yes, but not only that. The medical profession is pretty much locked in to the viral theory of AIDS. There is a lot of politics there. You have to understand that the only new money into biological research in recent years, new unmarked money, has been for Legionnaire's Disease and AIDS. As a result, laboratories are being built and careers are being made on this money. And the money is earmarked for research on the virus, not for the investigation of syphilis or of chemical immune suppression. Doctors who do not accept the official line on AIDS can find themselves in a lot of trouble.

HLC: That seems very plausible. And it wouldn't be the first time that purely scientific considerations had to take a back seat to economic imperatives. But tell me how you work with patients who have chronic inflammatory conditions, in order to promote normalcy?

JMcK: It's a little complicated to describe in an interview, but let me make a try. As a guideline for my method I take the thermal pattern of the body, meaning the pattern of temperature at various points on the surface and inside the body. This isn't the same as the patient's temperature. The temperature stays at 98.6 degrees plus or minus about three degrees, but the body's thermal pattern can have much greater temperature ranges. AIDS patients, and patients with chronic inflammatory conditions, have massive amounts of heat in their systems, and the whole thermal pattern is skewed upwards. We train people to normalize their thermal patterns by dietary and lifestyle changes, by intensive rehydration with deionized water, by mechanical cooling techniques, and in other ways. However, we do not use any drugs at all.

Essentially we are trying to cool down the body. If physiologic normalcy can be established, especially toward the cooler end of the normal thermodynamic, the microorganisms of opportunistic infections do not replicate. And the system then has a chance.

When it has been cooled down in this way, the body starts to behave as if it had competent immunity, even though it doesn't. It may not measure competent in terms of immunologic testing, but in terms of functional activity it behaves as if it had an immune system present. It buys some time. A non-reactive immune system starts to react. A patient who has been infected with syphilis, for instance, and whose serology is negative will frequently start to manifest positive serology.

This is all going to be necessary even if we do find a treatment for AIDS, because the survivors will still have to rebuild their immune systems. You have to be able to restore immunologic normalcy. Calm the system down.

Attitude also counts for a lot. Take the gay community, there is a lot of alcohol and drug abuse there, as well as sexual problems. Many of these people do not know how not to be victims. They have to learn how to take care of themselves, which usually they are not very good at. If they are going to survive, they have to stop defining themselves as victims. They have to take charge of their own lives.

The patient also needs some happiness, some laughter and enjoyment. All these improve the responsiveness of the immune-system. He has to start breathing and eating normally, listening to his body's signals. Studies in hospitals show that after surgery, if the individual is unstressed, recovery is 30 percent more rapid with 70 percent fewer complications.

I'll give you a case history: a male AIDS patient who had been treated for syphilis and had a 25-year history of drug and alcohol abuse. His serology was negative for syphilis, but after he had worked with me for a couple of months on immune-system stimulation, his serology became positive. In other words, his immune system was starting to kick in; it was now reacting to the syphilis infection which had never been entirely healed.

His internist didn't know what to do with this AIDS case

who had suddenly become a syphilis case. Sometimes when this happens the internist will just reject the finding of syphilis. He will say, "AIDS is a strange disease. We don't really know what is happening here, if this really is syphilis." But this internist was smart enough to send the patient to a syphilologist who treated him with benzathine G penicillin. He developed many of the symptoms of secondary syphilis, together with the roseola-like rash, which should have been a good sign. But his system was shot anyway, and in the end he died.

HLC: Have any of the medical organizations or authorities been supportive of what you are doing here?

JMcK: Since 1977 all of my hypotheses and methods have been on file with the American Medical Association and the American Cancer Society. I got in touch with the United States Food and Drug Administration too and said: "Here is what I am doing." They wrote back to me: "This isn't medicine, go away."

HLC: If they thought it wasn't medicine, then what was it?

JMcK: I don't know. Health maybe. About three years ago I contacted the Centers for Disease Control on the problem of identifying syphilis and syphilis antibodies in drug users and diseased people. Ninety-five percent of our AIDS clients had a history of syphilis, which meant they should have syphilis antibodies. Seventy percent of them didn't. If you can't find the syphilis, or any changes in antibody levels, no one will treat the patient for syphilis. The CDC told me to send them paired samples — meaning that you have a lab take a sample of blood from someone with syphilis, then you send half of it to the CDC and the other half to some diagnostic laboratory. After both have done the analysis, you compare them, and that way you have a baseline for a diagnosis of syphilis. Then the person gets the usual syphilis treatment, and when you think the patient is better, you take another set of paired samples and go through the same rigmarole all over again. What they really wanted me to do was to open up a venereal disease clinic to show how syphilis was evolving into AIDS.

HLC: I guess this would cost each patient a couple of thousand dollars.

JMcK: Yes, and it would take a long time. Furthermore, it would be a "one cause, one effect" model. And, at the end, maybe they would accept it and maybe not. We haven't got ten or twenty years to do that because we're looking at multiple assaults of disease and drugs — not one cause with one effect.

HLC: What they're really saying is "Get lost, babe," isn't it?

JMcK: It's a shame they can't just look at our findings with an open mind and get to work checking them out. Their problem is that they're following an old-fashioned model which is no longer applicable. They assume that the serological tests are always going to tell whether syphilis is or is not present, regardless of the present health and drug-use status of the patient. They assume that these tests are going to yield uniform and accurate readings, and they aren't. We have anomalies all over the place. We have men with known multiple histories of secondary syphilis presentations, who have been treated, who have no antibodies. And the doctors say: "It must have been a long time ago." And we say: "How about eight months, how about two years?" And so they say, "The patients must be very young." And we say, "No, no way, guys from 21 to 50." We may not exactly know the reason for these anomalies, but they exist.

About three years ago when I first started looking at this, I called the CDC, and I said, "Hi, if an individual is chemically immune-suppressed and contracts syphilis, would he necessarily produce antibodies to syphilis?" They said: "No." Then I asked, "If a person has AIDS and contracts syphilis, would he show antibodies to syphilis?" And they said, "No, not necessarily." I said, "Let me ask it another way: If a person is chemically immune-suppressed, and gets immune-suppressed from syphilis as well, he could have very bizarre symptoms but still have negative bloodwork?" And they said: "That's correct." So I asked: "Why aren't you surprised by these questions. When I called the California Department of Health, they started to get hysterical, because they had never thought of this before." And the CDC said: "Well, this isn't new." So I said, "What do you mean it isn't new?" And they said: "We've been getting calls for two years now from physicians who are treating men with AIDS whose symptoms are consistent with secondary syphilis but whose blood work is negative." So I asked: "Well, what are you doing about it?" And they said: "Nothing." And I said: "What are you *going* to do about it?" And they said: "Nothing."

It seems they had to have enough "evidence" that my hypothesis was correct before they would test. And their evidence consists of blood tests that I believe are invalid for the form of syphilis and the chemical immune suppression we are seeing in AIDS.

We've been looking at the full battery of syphilis tests: VDRL, RPR, MHA-TP, FTA-ABS, and even the TPI for two years now, and we see anomalies in all of them. Biopsies have been consistent with syphilis, and treponemes were even found in one patient.

But if you can't accurately test for syphilis with blood tests, if the standard treatments are just part of the cause, if, as a society, we have so overused chemicals that the very chemical makeup of the body is altered, then we are facing the failure of the biochemical approach to the treatment of disease.

HLC: I suppose they don't really know what to do about it.

JMcK: That's it. The rules of the game are changing. The old medical model is now turned against itself. But they keep relying on their belief system, they keep counting on syphilis to always show positive on the blood work, etc. etc. But this is no longer valid.

I have histories of gay men who have been on tetracycline for 18 years for the possibility of a pimple! I guarantee you their body chemistry isn't normal. I have guys with almost unlimited prescriptions for erythromycin, because every two or three weeks they will get a sore throat, and they'll take erythromycin for a few days to get rid of that sore throat. I guarantee you that this is an abuse of an antibiotic. I have individuals who, when they fill out their drug histories, give me three pages that are coded, to show which combinations of drugs they were on in any given period. Often they were taking two or three prescribed drugs — valium, librium, erythromycin — plus designer drugs (you know the gay community invented the designer drug*), amyl nitrite, butyl nitrite, uppers, downers, and they would give me a whole coding. We are talking about a community where drugs are rampant.

We don't have any idea of what their body chemistry is any more. And we don't know how much of the general population is in the same kind of chemical distortion.

How about the Vietnam vets? The Veterans' Administration has said that 20–30 percent of the returning vets brought back with them a form of hepatitis which they call "non-specific AB hepatitis." There's no medical treatment for it, and so they just walk around with inflamed livers (which is what hepatitis is). The liver is a very important part of the immune system. When the liver is off, you don't have the same reactions, don't make the same antibodies. What does chronic liver inflammation do to the immune response to syphilis? There are a lot of returned vets in the San Francisco area.

I am in contact with the companies who make the lab-test kits. They know perfectly well that if the individual is taking any kind of therapeutic or other drug, or has a chronic inflammatory disease such as hepatitis or nephritis, and then gets syphilis, the blood work isn't necessarily going to show it. There can be false negatives all over the place, with a rampaging syphilis infection.

So I went back and called the CDC and asked, "How can we screen? I mean, this is making me crazy. I have men here

---

*"Designer drugs" are recreational drugs that have been chemically altered just enough to make them technically unregulated.

with a history of syphilis, but the blood work doesn't show anything; they have no antibodies." Their doctors in San Francisco say that can't be. They say, "I know this patient, I've treated this patient for syphilis. It can't be. He's got to have the antibodies. I won't give him the antibody test." So I say, "Why not. It's a cheap test. Why not give it?" The reason is they're sure the result will be positive; they *know* it will be positive. Because they've never seen an individual in the gay community with syphilis who went negative on the antibody test. But the doctors are wrong. Seventy percent of the men in my program with a known history of syphilis have no antibodies to it.

I had one man who came in from Toronto who had a known history of secondary syphilis. He came down. He was tested, and no antibodies. I showed him how to take care of himself. I worked with him. He went back to Canada and saw his doctor there who was an AIDS specialist; he said, of course, you have antibodies. So the doctor sent him to his own lab, and there too he came up with no antibodies. So the doctor hemmed and hawed and said maybe it was a bad day at the lab. So two or three months later he went and got tested again (as I had told him to do) because now he was showing secondary syphilis presentation, with the rash. I told him to go and make them examine him based on signs and symptoms and ask if it wasn't a syphilis presentation. The people at the clinic said it was secondary syphilis. And they took a blood test, and this time he showed antibodies, because he was on my program that was coaching his immune system to behave as if it was normal (but they wouldn't treat him for syphilis, anyway, because the doctor wanted him to go on an anti-viral drug program for AIDS).

I have men in the gay community with 5000 sexual partners a year. And that isn't even the record. They will say to one another, "How many would you say so-and-so had? . . . Maybe 12,000 . . . a really busy man." I will ask them if they ever had sex with a Vietnam vet, and they will answer, "I know a lot of faceless men."

HLC: Well, what does all this mean?

JMcK: It means that with AIDS we are in a new ballgame, and the medical profession should realize this. In recent years the doctors have taken a highly defensive stand in terms of their legal position vis-a-vis the rest of society. There is an element in the AMA (and in the mass media) which wants to go after every doctor or health worker who is against a chemotherapeutic cure for AIDS. They polarize society against everyone who is offering any other kind of insight into the nature of the disease or the nature of the community being treated. There has to be truce between the medical profession, the media, and everyone else for the sake of the AIDS patients themselves.

For instance, over at San Francisco General Hospital there is a group of long-term AIDS survivors—who have survived three or four years. The docs themselves will tell you that those who survive are the ones who at some point came to the decision to make behavioral, lifestyle, and emotional changes. They've decided to take control over their own lives. They refuse to rely on physicians telling them what to do. Everyone knows that is true. But a physician at this hospital has stated publicly, "If I tried to go around and advise AIDS patients that they had to do this, I would be accused of quackery."

HLC: Can you tell us something about your own results?

JMcK: I haven't been entirely successful. Out of the 32 AIDS cases I started with initially, 11 have died, so I am running about a 30 percent loss rate. But the men who are left are healthier. Some have already survived six or seven years.

HLC: What kind of diagnosis do you do? I mean, how do you know when they are better or worse?

JMcK: I don't do any diagnosing. They have to have a physician.

HLC: How do you know they have AIDS, then?

JMcK: From the physician's diagnosis, and they fill out a lengthy medical history form.

HLC: And after you've had them in your program for a while, do they go back to the doctor and be checked again?

JMcK: Yes, the doctors check the T-cells, etc. But, of course, these studies of T-cells are not necessarily accurate. We don't always know what the T-cells are actually measuring. They can fluctuate radically. A virus infection, such as Epstein-Barr virus, can off the T-cells. So can a fight with your mother. When there is an alteration in T-cell ratios, all it means is that there is some kind of infection or alarm. So I rely more on other factors. For instance, they shouldn't have any secondary infections. They should feel better. Their other symptoms should disappear. Sometimes they will put on weight. Or, if they don't put on weight, you have to understand why. I have a guy who has just opened a second business. For six weeks he was running around like a maniac, and he started losing weight. So he comes to me and says, "What should I do, I'm losing weight?" So I told him that in his circumstances that was entirely normal and that he should slow down, rest, and go play.

HLC: Is anyone you know treating AIDS with penicillin?

JMcK: Yes, there are three or four physicians in the Bay area, the same number in Los Angeles, and maybe six or seven in New York. Up to now six of our clients have received this treatment. Four died, but two are starting to look like successes.

HLC: What do you think is the reason for the failures?

JMcK: Two of the failures had a history of drug abuse, one very seriously, one less so. For the other two the treatment may just have come too late, or the treatment may not work in all cases.

HLC: Do you think that those who have just syphilis in the background, and not a history of severe drug abuse, might respond better to penicillin treatment?

JMcK: That's a definite possibility. Of our two successes so far, one had a history of no drug use, while the other had only taken small doses of ampicillin. Dierig in Germany has about six successes, and he feels that all have minimal histories of drug involvement. Of course, if the AIDS patient is *treated* with medicinal drugs of the wrong kind, this could also skew the case and make it later incurable by penicillin.

HLC: Have the insurance companies shown any interest in what you are doing?

JMcK: Yes, some of them have even reimbursed my guys for working with me, because their medical bills are *less* than what other people cost.

HLC: What would you like to say in conclusion?

JMcK: We have to be willing to help people rebuild their lives, as well as their bodies, once the syphilis is redressed. Until physicians and researchers realize that they are in a technological bind in diagnosing chemically immune-suppressed or disease-suppressed syphilis, our methods can only buy a little time for people with AIDS. If they're lucky, they'll have enough immunity to react to the syphilis so it can be diagnosed. Until it is diagnosed by a physician, it can't be treated. And even if treated, what we have now may not cure it. AIDS is simply a new face, a new disguise, a new chemical environment for syphilis — an old and infinitely resourceful enemy.

We have to reevaluate our methods and our medicines. We have to marshall all our resources, or we shall know another Middle Ages, where wave after wave of disease nearly destroyed Europe. We should keep in mind the saying that "Those who do not learn from history get to repeat it!"

Appendix B

Interview with Stephen Caiazza, M.D.

Stephen S. Caiazza, M.D. was the first American physician to start treating AIDS patients with penicillin. This interview was recorded in June, 1987.

HLC: Dr. Caiazza, why don't you start off by telling me how you came to the idea of testing your patients for syphilis.

SC: I have been working with AIDS patients, to all intents and purposes, since I started my practice in 1982. I soon came to realize that there was something screwy, because I was hardly seeing any cases of syphilis. While there was an exponential increase in AIDS/ARC/HIV infection, I was only getting one or two cases of syphilis per year. I have one of the biggest gay practices in Manhattan, and I thought it strange that syphilis was going away, while AIDS was increasing logarithmically, especially since they are both transmitted in the same way.

I thought, Lord, I've got a large gay practice in Manhattan, I should be seeing more syphilis. In addition, a few of my patients with full-blown AIDS would sometimes come up with a positive VDRL or some other serological result indicating infection with syphilis. Those patients I treated in the standard way for syphilis, i.e., with penicillin, and while I was treating them, their AIDS got better. This was just a coincidence, I thought, something I wasn't looking for.

Then I had a couple of patients with very unusual lesions — some in the throat, which the ear-nose-throat guy couldn't figure out, some in the gall-bladder, which no one could figure out either. So I began treating them for syphilis, and those lesions melted away. So I began to suspect that there was some confusion here between AIDS and syphilis, but I decided it was just test interference.

The next big thing that happened was in September, 1986. I had just finished being part of a big behind-the-scenes campaign to get AZT released. The FDA relaxed some of its guidelines, and I figured that was going to take care of the AIDS problem (I was wrong there). I was feeling tired and sick, and figured my work was done anyway, so I announced my retirement. And I was lying on my sofa at home, feeling a little depressed, when the telephone rang, and it was Joan McKenna calling from Switzerland. She asked me, "I understand you're interested in the role of syphilis in AIDS." I said, "Yes." She said, "Have you ever heard of Dr. Dierig in Augsburg?" I said, "I've never heard of Augsburg, let alone Dr. Dierig." Anyway, she told me about him, so I called Dierig on the phone, and we talked for maybe an hour.

Within 48 hours I was on the plane to Augsburg. I brought a whole bunch of my clinical data there. We sat down one night in a bar there, together with his colleague, Urban Waldthaler. We compared numbers, and we said, "Holy Christ, there's something going on that we had never figured. Syphilis is playing some kind of major role."

HLC: So Dierig had come on this independently?

SC: Not only independently, but he was ahead of me. We were paralleling. But he had made a leap that I hadn't made — to causality.

94

Joan McKenna joined us there, by the way, and we had a talk. She had this program for AIDS patients in Berkeley and was doing ordinary background investigations on them, and she found a lot of syphilis there. We were all paralleling each other.

I then went back to the US. I had frozen sera from about twenty of my patients who had died. All dead. I kept the sera frozen, packed it in dry ice, which is a major production, got back on a plane, and went back to Germany. That's when we tested my sera with the VDRL and other syphilis serological tests.

I also had some frozen cerebrospinal fluid from patients who had died of "squash rot" from AIDS, and there also we turned up hordes of syphilis treponemes. By the way, I had deliberately brought, by and large, people who had a negative history of syphilis. I wanted to avoid the whole can of worms of "Well, they had syphilis before. That's why your tests are positive." I intentionally selected fourteen or eighteen out of twenty cases who had never had syphilis, or so we thought. So even if we only got a positive FTA, that was still important data.

I had one incredible patient who had died of AIDS encephalopathy with essentially no brain left.* He had received a tremendous workup, even checking for Kreutzfeld-Jakob disease. This cerebrospinal fluid was very strongly positive for syphilis, but his VDRL was negative or non-reactive. And, as far as he or anyone else knew, *the man had never had syphilis.*

I then came back to America and closed down my operation here. I went on sabbatical. Also I was not feeling well. Not only I was depressed from having buried so many patients and friends from 1982 to 1986, hundreds of people you identify with, all young men. But I was also coming down with

---

*"Encephalopathy": a kind of brain inflammation, similar to an encephalitis.

the first stages of AIDS and didn't know it.

The story is as follows. I knew I had to be AIDS-virus positive because of the many puncture wounds from hypodermics while treating AIDS patients, but I had never had syphilis. When I went to Germany on the second trip, we needed a negative control for our experiments. I said I am the perfect negative control. We tested my serum for HIV, and, sure enough, the virus was there in large quantities. But there was zero syph, no evidence of *T. pallidum*. So they could use my serum as a control.

So I went back to the US with that knowledge. I was HIV positive because of the puncture wounds, but by history, and by a thorough serological examination, no syphilis. But then, before leaving for my third trip to Germany, and without telling Dierig or Waldthaler, I deliberately inoculated myself with syphilis.

HLC: Wow!

SC: Well, big deal, syphilis, so what.

HLC: When was this?

SC: Mid-October to late October, 1986. They didn't know it. I inoculated myself with syphilis. Then I went back to Germany in the second week of December, 1986, where Dierig was having trouble with a couple of patients and consulted with him on a few tight clinical spots. Then I suddenly started to get sick: tremendous colitis, horrible depression, inability to concentrate. Couldn't sit still, terrible memory for recent events. It was almost like an encephalopathy.

I was still commuting back and forth to Germany, and before I would get on the plane, Dierig would give me a milligram of atropine subcutaneously so I wouldn't have to spend the whole flight in the toilet. I had this intractable colitis. We didn't know why. Just to get across the Atlantic without a major diarrhoea number was hard to manage.

That's when I told Dierig, "Guess what I've done." And I'll never forget. He turned to me and said, in his broken English, "My friend, this time I think you go too far!" I got sick as a dog.

HLC: Let me clarify a couple of points. If you were doing this experiment on yourself, why did you let it run so long. How long were you prepared to let it run?

SC: The problem was we didn't know what the incubation time was. I inoculated myself in October, got really sick in mid-November, had to keep shooting myself up with atropine, and my mind was starting to go real bad at that point, I could tell. I had assumed I was dealing with a 6-month or 1-year incubation period, but in fact the incubation period was maybe ten days or two weeks.

So I went back to Germany thinking maybe this was the end, and they hooked me up to an IV, and I started getting penicillin by vein. It was a very stormy course, because we kept having these incredible problems. I had brought all my computers with me, and I was planning to do some more work. But for various reasons we kept having to move from place to place.

One time we were out driving at 3 A.M., and this other car, with a very skillful driver, comes up behind and almost runs us off the road. There was never any explanation.

Then another time I am at a hotel in Augsburg, and it was the day after Christmas, 1986. I hadn't been able to walk for two weeks, I was so blown away. So I finally get up, leave my room, close the door, lock it, and head for the elevators. At that point I am hit on the head from behind with a club or some blunt object, fall down unconscious on the floor, and wake up a few minutes later all covered with blood. When I fell, I hit an artery, a pumper, on something, and it took fifteen sutures in my forehead to sew it up.

I have pictures of the hotel corridor, all covered with blood.

I was also totally non compos mentis. Dierig came in about that time, found me wandering around all bloody, and thought I was drunk from the way I was staggering. He came up and said, "My God, your head's busted open, you're bleeding like a pig." All I wanted to do was to go back into the room and close the door, but he arranged for one of his friends to have me sutured at the hospital, got me out of the hotel, and I stayed with him and his family for the duration.

HLC: Who do you think did this?

SC: I have no idea. A full report was filed on December 27 with the Augsburg police, but the guy who did it has never been found. All I know is that we later met a lawyer there and told him this story. It turned out that his specialty is industrial espionage. Dierig was telling him about it in Deutsch. Then he looks at both of us and says, "Gentlemen, are you aware that forty percent of all pharmaceuticals for the Western world are produced in West Germany?"

We looked stupid and said, no, we didn't know that.

And he said, "Gentlemen, if what you're telling me is true, then you're both in great danger." That's as much as I know.

Maybe I got hit in the head because somebody didn't like my looks. How do I know?

HLC: What you're really suggesting is that people are making a lot of money out of AZT and these other medicines, and nobody wants to bring penicillin in to treat AIDS.

SC: Yeah, if our theory's right, nobody's going to make much money out of treating AIDS.

HLC: Is penicillin a patented medicine?

SC: No, its generic. Anybody that has a proper license can manufacture it.

HLC: And it's as cheap as dirt, isn't it.

SC: It ain't so expensive. Compared with AZT that costs, what is it, $10,000 per patient per year, we're talking two or three hundred dollars. It's pennies. Compared to the recommended AIDS medicine, we're talking nickels and dimes.

HLC: OK, so you continued with your treatment and recovered from it?

SC: Yes, we had to do that experiment. There was no way I was going to come back to the United States and subject my *patients* to this treatment without knowing about it first. While I was ninety percent sure that penicillin would be curative, I wasn't ninety-nine percent sure. I had to do that experiment. It was crucial.

HLC: Well, it was a very heroic thing to do.

SC: Ahh, it wasn't so heroic. Everyone likes to play Walter Reed once in a while. Until we controlled it, we simply didn't know what was what. But what is maybe most interesting is that we never found any traces of the treponemes in me, even with a spinal tap. I had AIDS-virus in every orifice we tested, but no trace of the treponemes.

They had to have been there. The doc who injected me took the treponemes himself from a patient of mine with virgin syphilis. Then he injected me with them. I don't know what the dose was, but I got a wonderful skin lesion out of it. And I got as sick as a dog. But we never found evidence of syphilis in me, which proves the other point I've been trying to make. You've got to go by clinical insight. You can't depend on the laboratory findings all the time.

HLC: So you mean to say you were never able to demonstrate the presence of treponemes.

SC: That's right, including all of the serological and other lab tests you can think of.

HLC: What is the reason for that?

SC: We speculate that when there's AIDS-virus aboard, there's interference. The tests we use to find the AIDS-virus assume a functioning immune system. Syphilis impairs the immune system more than AIDS-virus does. So when you add the impairment with AIDS-virus, is it so ridiculous to assume that maybe the immune system simply can't function.

HLC: Clearly the AIDS virus and the treponeme together cause a huge amount of confusion in the body.

SC: Yes, they mess up all the diagnostic tests completely.

HLC: OK, so now you're back from Germany, back in the mainstream, so what do you do now?

SC: I came back to New York January 9, got my bearings for a month or so, did some more writing and networking. April 14 or 15 we opened the office again, and we've been going like gangbusters ever since.

HLC: What treatment are you using?

SC: Aqueous penicillin is best, but it has to be given intravenously in the hospital. Now, if I had a real sickie, in the hospital, of course I'd use aqueous. But my practice now is entirely with outpatients. I can't take 500,000 people in Manhattan, put them in the hospital, shove an IV in them, and keep them there for 3 weeks.

The usual regimen I use on my out-patients is to go three weeks with benzathine penicillin, the kind I said earlier not to use, because it doesn't cross the blood-brain barrier and go into the brain, but it's perfectly good for the periphery. So if a guy has a shot immune system or other peripheral symptoms, and isn't suicidal, I zap him real good, taking care of the periphery. Week four I give doxycycline, which can cross the blood-brain barrier, and he takes it by mouth for several months. That hits not only the periphery but the brain as well. I've had to come up with this regimen simply as a logistical necessity.

We don't use amoxycillin because it doesn't cross the blood-brain barrier.

Now the English will take someone and give him daily injections for three weeks. I could do that too, but, No. 1, that's also logistically difficult and, No. 2, show me the patient who will let you do that to him — a daily injection for 20 days!

HLC: Now, can you say how many patients you've treated this way?

SC: About three dozen.

HLC: How many of them are showing signs of improvement?

SC: Well, all of them. But it's still very preliminary, as they've only been in treatment for a few weeks.

HLC: Have you attempted to deal with the authorities on this?

SC: Yes, in early February I met with Dr. Stephen Joseph, Health Commissioner of the City of NY, and presented him with the data, and I said, "There will be a lot of arguments over whether we are right or Robert Gallo is right, but no one will deny the following. In New York City there is a reservoir of untreated syphilis. Dierig and Caiazza are saying that this reservoir is huge, essentially the same size as the AIDS reservoir. But current wisdom holds to the contrary view, that the reservoir exists but isn't so big. Let's ignore how big the reservoir is, but go out and treat it properly, and then let's see what happens to the AIDS incidence. Even if we're wrong, and our treatments don't have any impact on the AIDS incidence, at least we will reduce the incidence of syphilis. I don't expect you're going to believe us, because this is very unorthodox. But let us do our little trick, make us do it again in a fishbowl, and you be the judge and analyze the data."

Dr. Joseph replied with the comment that it would be "inappropriate for us to fund your research at this time. . . . I have asked the Department to pursue this question, internally, further." He enclosed an internal memorandum from Dr. Rand Stoneburner, Director of AIDS Research for the New York Dept. of Health. It said: (1) Caiazza doesn't know how to interpret data, (2) those people he claims had syphilis, despite the medical history to the contrary, well, the histories are wrong, and (3) he's probably lying anyway; how do we know he's telling the truth?

HLC: The authorities always seem to take the view that you have to prove everything first before they will even consider an idea. They're like the man from Missouri who says, "Show me." They automatically assume that you have the burden of proof. Why should you with limited resources have to be making the demonstration and not them? After all, the public is paying them to check out every possibility? They are living on our tax dollars. Seems to me they might shoulder some of the burden of proof themselves provided the hypothesis is a reasonable one. People don't usually think about this aspect.

SC: You're right. I was proposing an interesting hypothesis to them, and they just turned it down flat. As I wrote to Dr. Joseph later, "You took a no-lose solution — and lost."

HLC: So, was that the end of your efforts to persuade the New York authorities?

SC: No, I then wrote to the State Health Department and got a relatively encouraging reply from Dr. George T. DiFerdinando, Jr. in Albany, asking precisely what we wanted to do. I wrote back in June, but there hasn't yet been any answer.

I have had better luck with the federal government. In the late spring I met Dr. Robert Redfield, who is head of AIDS research for the Walter Reed Army Medical Center in Washington. I explained all of this to him, and he was very excited. He said, "Well, if you're talking central nervous system, you may be right, because retroviruses can't do to the central nervous system what we're seeing here. In fact," he said, "I'll go back and talk to Ed Tramont about it." And now Ed Tramont has written an editorial in last week's *New England Journal of Medicine* about AIDS and syphilis, which is very exciting. So Redfield was supportive.*

In the meantime I decided to go to the lay press, the *New York Native, Penthouse,* and others, so the word has gone out, and people are talking about this theory now. This reminds me of a funny story. I had to call a physician colleague the other day who also treats AIDS patients, and he said to me

---

*See "Syphilis in the AIDS Era" (editorial). *New England Journal of Medicine* 316:25 (1987), 1600–1601. See, also, Donald R. Jones *et al.,* "Alteration in the Natural History of Neurosyphilis by Concurrent Infection with the Human Immunodeficiency Virus." *New England Journal of Medicine* 316:25 (1987), 1569–1572. Carol Dawn Berry *et al.,* "Neurologic Relapse After Benzathine Penicillin Therapy for Secondary Syphilis in a Patient with HIV Infection." *New England Journal of Medicine* 316:25 (1987), 1587–1589.

on the telephone, "Caiazza, you are public enemy number one."

I said, "Jeff, what's wrong."

He says, "The phone doesn't stop ringing. All our patients (he's in a group) want to know if we've checked them for syphilis. And they all ask if we use 'Dr. Caiazza's technique.'"

And I said, "But Jeffrey, isn't that nice." He said, "We're putting out a contract on you."

HLC: Why is he so hostile to using "Dr. Caiazza's technique?"

SC: That's just what I asked him, and he said, "It's because you're wrong."

And I said, "But Jeffrey, are you sure I'm wrong?"

And he said, "Of course you're wrong, everyone knows that a virus causes this disease, and anyone who questions the viral origin of AIDS needs a lumbar puncture himself."

HLC: You don't suppose it's because they're making much more money treating with AZT?

SC: As far as the industry is concerned, there is no question in my mind that it is a financial question. If I had announced discovering a new strain of *T. pallidum* that can be treated only with this very expensive new medicine that is under license to Hoffman-Laroche, I don't think I would have any trouble at all. But because I talk about penicillin and doxycycline which are generic drugs, I am meeting with a lot of resistance.

That's for the industry. As far as my colleagues are concerned it's something else. I remember what I went through. I remember lying in that bed in Augsburg and existing only due to the kindness of strangers, but feeling much better, and looking up at that IV and saying to myself, "My God, I'm a doctor, and I've buried all those people," and their faces kind of came to me at 3 o'clock in the morning. "I've buried all those people," I thought, "and I missed that diagnosis which I shouldn't have missed and, mainly, that I could have done something about." That's really horrible. You have to go through your own catharsis before you can face that. We doctors in New York are all exhausted. We're all working as hard as we can. And it's not wonderful to wake up one morning and say to yourself, "You missed a treatable disease." That's hard.

In New York State doctors can, in fact, dispense, but I don't know any doctors who are dispensing AZT. They give the patient a prescription. So they don't make money on the prescriptions. I hope that no one is motivated that way, anyway, even though there are plenty of swine in the medical profession. No, it's not that. It's more complex. By and large doctors are honorable people. We want our patients to get better.

And there are a lot of doctors who don't want to deal with AIDS anyway. I'm sure if you went out there and said, I have a magic pill, and all your AIDS problems will go away, they would say, "How do I get it?"

HLC: Is that all?

SC: That's about it. It's an unfolding story.

Notes

Introduction

1. N. Dozier *et al.*, "Acquired Immune Deficiency Syndrome and the Management of Associated Opportunistic Infections." *Drug Intelligence and Clinical Pharmacy* 17 (1983), 798–807. R. E. Stahl *et al.*, "AIDS: a Medical Conundrum." *J. Cutaneous Pathology* 10 (1983), 550–558.

2. M. W. Vogt *et al.*, "Isolation of HTLV-III/LAV From Cervical Secretions of Women at Risk for AIDS." *The Lancet* (March 8, 1986), 525–527. C. F. Wofsy *et al.*, "Isolation of AIDS-Associated Retrovirus from Genital Secretions of Women with Antibodies to the Virus." *The Lancet* (March 8, 1986), 527–529. "New Link Found in Spreading of Immune Illness." *Washington Post,* January 7, 1983, A-3.

3. Centers for Disease Control, Center for Infectious Diseases. AIDS WEEKLY SURVEILLANCE REPORT — UNITED STATES AIDS PROGRAM. June 15, 1987 (unpublished).

4. Jamie Murphy, "Gloom in the Palais des Congres." *Time,* July 7, 1986, 51. Susan Okie, "Heterosexual AIDS May Surge, Koop Says." *Washington Post,* April 21, 1987, A-4.

5. *Loc. cit.* William Kronholm, "Commission on AIDS Needed, Says US Agency." *Boston Globe,* June 13, 1986, 1.

6. *Loc. cit.* Robert Pear, "Tenfold Increase in AIDS Death Toll is Expected by '91." *New York Times,* June 13, 1986, A-1.

7. Lawrence K. Altman, "Global Program Aims to Combat AIDS 'Disaster.'" *New York Times*, November 21, 1986. 1.

8. T. C. Quinn *et al.*, "AIDS in Africa: An Epidemiologic Paradigm." *Science* 234 (1986), 955–963. William F. Buckley, Jr., "What Can We *Do* About AIDS?" *Washington Post*, April 23, 1987, A–23.

Chapter I — Microbe or Host Organism?

1. Claudia Wallis, "AIDS: A Growing Threat," *Time*, August 12, 1985, 40–47. Jonathan Lieberson, "The Reality of AIDS," *New York Review of Books*, January 16, 1986, 43–48.

2. James W. Curran *et al.*, "The Epidemiology of AIDS: Current Status and Future Prospects." *Science* 229 (1985), 1352–1357. R. E. Stahl, *et al.*, *op. cit.*

3. Vincent T. DeVita, Jr., Samuel Hellman, Steven A. Rosenberg, *AIDS: Etiology, Diagnosis, Treatment, and Prevention.* Philadelphia: Lippincott, 1985.

4. F. Denis *et al.*, "Prevalence of Human T-Lymphotropic Retroviruses Type III (HIV) and Type IV in Ivory Coast." *The Lancet* (February 21, 1987), 408–411. Lawrence K. Altman, "Third AIDS Virus Found in Sweden." *New York Times*, November 20, 1986, A-24. "Second AIDS Virus Said to be Deadly." *New York Times*, November 8, 1986, 1. Robert Steinbrook, "Scientist Warns of Threat from New AIDS Virus." *Los Angeles Times*, November 7, 1986, 1.

5. Lawrence K. Altman, "How AIDS Researchers Strive for Virus Proof." *New York Times*, October 23, 1984, C-3.

6. J. W. Curran, *op. cit.* R. E. Stahl, *op. cit.* Peter H. Duesberg, "Retroviruses as Carcinogens and Pathogens: Expectations and Reality." *Cancer Research* 47 (1987), 1199–1220.

7. Peter H. Duesberg, *op. cit.*

Chapter II — The Syphilis Connection

1. E. G. Clark and N. Danbolt, "The Oslo Study of the Natural Course of Untreated Syphilis." *Medical Clinics of North America* 48:3 (1964), 613–623.

2. Loyd Thompson, *Syphilis*. Philadelphia and New York: Lea and Febiger, 1920, 29, 31.

3. P. D. Woolley and A. J. Anderson, "Prevalence of Undiagnosed Syphilis in the Elderly" (letter). *The Lancet* (November 1, 1986), 1034.

4. William F. Danehower, "Penicillin Fallout and Infectious Syphilis." *Medical Clinics of North America* 48:3 (1964), 747–753.

5. *Loc. cit.*

6. Rudolph H. Kampmeier *et al.*, "A Survey of 251 Patients with Acute Syphilis Treated in the Collaborative Penicillin Study of 1943–1950," *Sexually Transmitted Diseases* 8:4 (1981), 266–279.

7. A. L. Schroeter *et al.*, "Treatment for Early Syphilis and Reactivity of Serologic Tests." *JAMA* 221:5 (1972), 471–476. "Congenital Syphilis — United States, 1983–1985." *Morbidity and Mortality Weekly Report* 35: 43, 1986.

8. J. J. Potterat *et al.*, "Serologic Markers as Indicators of Sexual Orientation in AIDS Virus-Infected Men." (letter) *JAMA* 256:6 (1986), 712.

9. Michael Specter, "Fear of AIDS Cited as Syphilis Rate Declines." *Washington Post*, August 10, 1985, A-1. Lewis M. Drusin, "Syphilis: Clinical Manifestations, Diagnosis, and Treatment." *Urologic Clinics of North America* 11:1 (1984), 121–130.

10. Harold W. Jaffe, *et al.*, "National Case-Control Study of Kaposi's Sarcoma and *Pneumocystis carinii* Pneumonia in Homosexual Men: Part 1, Epidemiologic Results." *Annals of Internal Medicine* 99:2 (1983), 145–151. Martha F. Rogers, *et al.*, "Part 2, Laboratory Results." *Ibid.*, 151–158.

11. Mary E. Guinan *et al.*, "Heterosexual and Homosexual Patients with the Acquired Immunodeficiency Syndrome," *Annals of Internal Medicine* 100 (1984), 213–218.

12. CDC, AIDS WEEKLY SURVEILLANCE REPORT — UNITED STATES AIDS PROGRAM. June 15, 1987. M. Robert-Guroff *et al.*, "Prevalence of Antibodies to HTLV-I, -II, and -III in Intravenous Drug Abusers from an AIDS Epidemic Region." *JAMA* 255:22 (1986), 3133–3137.

13. CDC, AIDS WEEKLY SURVEILLANCE REPORT — UNITED STATES AIDS PROGRAM. June 15, 1987.

14. Mary E. Guinan *et al.*, *op. cit.*

15. Jonathan Cohen, "AIDS: A Review." *British Journal of Hospital Medicine* 31:4 (1984), 250–254, 258–259.

16. K. Weismann, J. H. Sindrup, and G. L. Wantzin, "Syphilisprofilen hos LAV/HTLV-III-antistof-positive og -negative homoseksuelle maend." *Ugeskr. Laeger* 148:14 (1986), 823–825.

17. Harold W. Jaffe *et al.*, *op. cit.*

18. J. J. McKenna *et al.*, "Unmasking AIDS: Chemical Immunosuppression and Seronegative Syphilis." *Medical Hypotheses* 21:4 (1986), 421–430.

19. Raymond A. Smego, *et al.*, "Secondary Syphilis Masquerading as AIDS in a Young Gay Male." *North Carolina Medical Journal* 45 (1984), 253–254.

20. J. A. Stroh, "The 'Great Imitator' Keeps Up with the Times." *Hospital Practice*, November 15, 1986, 33–38.

21. N. Dozier *et al.*, *op. cit.* P. M. Feorino *et al.*, "Transfusion-Associated Acquired Immunodeficiency Syndrome: Evidence for Persistent Infection in Blood Donors." *New England Journal of Medicine* 312:20 (1985), 1293–1296. "Surveillance of Hemophilia-Associated Acquired Immunodeficiency Syndrome." *Morbidity and Mortality Weekly Reports*, 35:40, 1986.

22. J. J. Van Der Sluis, *et al.*, "Transfusion Syphilis, Survival of *Treponema pallidum* in Stored Donorblood." *Vox sanguinis* 49 (1985), 390–399.

23. J. J. McKenna *et al.*, *op. cit.* J. J. Thompson *et al.*, "Immunoregulatory Properties of Serum from Patients with Different Stages of Syphilis." *British Journal of Venereal Diseases* 56 (1980) 210–217.

24. "Congenital Syphilis — United States, 1983–1985." *MMWR* 35:43 (1986).

25. N. Dozier *et al.*, *op. cit.*

26. Loyd Thompson, *op. cit.*, 27.

27. P. C. Desmangles, "Controle des Maladies Veneriennes en Haiti." *Bulletin de l'Association Medicale Haitienne* 8: 3–4 (1956).

28. J. W. Pape *et al.*, "Characteristics of the Acquired Immunodeficiency Syndrome (AIDS) in Haiti." *New England Journal of Medicine* 309:16 (1983), 945–950.

29. F. Denis *et al.*, *op. cit.* Thomas C. Quinn *et al.*, *op. cit.*

30. Peter Piot *et al.*, "Acquired Immunodeficiency Syndrome in a Heterosexual Population in Zaire." *The Lancet* (July 14, 1984), 65–69.

31. Philippe Van de Perre *et al.*, "Acquired Immunodeficiency Syndrome in Rwanda." *The Lancet* (July 14, 1984), 62–65.

32. Blaine Harden, "Uganda Battles AIDS Epidemic." *Washington Post*, June 2, 1986, A-1.

33. A.E.J. Masawe, "Serological Tests for Syphilis in Uganda," *East African Medical Journal* 47:12 (1970), 673–680.

34. A.E.J. Masawe *et al.*, "Unusual Behavior of Serological Tests for Syphilis in Ugandan Africans." *British Journal of Venereal Diseases* 48 (1972) 345–349.

35. P. R. Mason *et al.*, "The Serological Diagnosis of Syphilis." *The Central African Journal of Medicine* 31:10 (1985), 192–193.

36. S. A. Ahmed *et al.*, "Prevalence of Syphilis in South Sudan." *J. Com. Dis.* 17:3 (1985), 251.

37. *Loc. cit.*

38. Thomas C. Quinn *et al.*, "Serologic and Immunologic Studies in Patients with AIDS in North America and Africa." *JAMA* 257:19 (1987), 2617–2621. Editorial: "Africa and the Biology of Human Immunodeficiency Virus." *JAMA* 257:19 (1987), 2632–2633.

39. N. Clumeck *et al.*, "Acquired Immunodeficiency Syndrome in African Patients." *New England Journal of Medicine* 310:8 (1984), 492–497.

40. J. K. Kreiss *et al.*, "AIDS Virus Infection in Nairobi Prostitutes." *New England Journal of Medicine* 314:7 (1986), 414–418.

41. F. Denis *et al.*, *op. cit.*

42. Thomas C. Quinn *et al.*, "Serologic and Immunologic Studies in Patients with AIDS in North America and Africa."

43. Editorial: "Kaposi's Sarcoma." *The Lancet* (February 10, 1973), 300–301.

44. S. M. Bluefarb, *Kaposi's Sarcoma* (Springfield, Thomas, 1957), 36, 130. Philippe van de Perre *et al., op. cit.*

45. Lawrence Altman, "Linking AIDS to Africa Provokes Bitter Debate." *New York Times*, November 21, 1985, A-1.

46. Lewis M. Drusin, *op. cit.*

47. E. Foged *et al.*, "Biological False Positives to Serological Tests for Syphilis in Herpes Genitalis." *Annals of Clinical Research* 17 (1985), 71–72.

48. A. Luger *et al.*, "Recent Observations on the Serology of Syphilis." *British Journal of Venereal Diseases* 56 (1980), 12–16.

49. M. Gibowski *et al.*, "Non-Specific Positive Test Results to Syphilis in Dermatological Diseases." *British Journal of Venereal Diseases* 56 (1980), 17–19. See, also, articles in *Journal of the American Venereal Disease Association* 3:1 (1976).

50. A. Luger *et al., op. cit.* Sidney Olansky, "Serodiagnosis of Syphilis." *Medical Clinics of North America* 56:5 (1972), 1145–1150.

51. J. Lawton Smith and Charles W. Israel, "The Presence of Spirochetes in Late Seronegative Syphilis." *JAMA* 199:13 (1967), 980–984. J. J. McKenna *et al., op. cit.*

52. P. Collart and M. Poitevin, "Is Penicillin Therapy Always Infallible in Syphilis?" *J. Clin. Neuro-Ophthalm.* 2 (1982), 77–83. P. Frederick Sparling, "Diagnosis and Treatment of Syphilis." *New England Journal of Medicine* 284:12 (1971), 642–653.

53. Editorial: "Treatment of Primary and Secondary Syphilis: Defining Failure at Three- and Six-Month Follow-up." *JAMA* 257:3 (1987), 359–360.

54. Personal communication from Stephen S. Caiazza, M.D.

55. Personal communication from Stephen S. Caiazza, M.D.

56. Editorial: "Syphilis in the AIDS Era." *New England Journal of Medicine* 316:25 (1987), 1600–1601.

Chapter III — Syphilis Suppression During the Great Postwar Penicillin Fallout

1. H. H. Volan, "Diagnosis of Early Syphilis." *New York State Journal of Medicine* (1966), 2908–2912.

2. R. A. Smego *et al.*, *op. cit.* Lewis M. Drusin, "Syphilis: Clinical Manifestations, Diagnosis, and Treatment." G. T. Strickland, *Hunter's Tropical Medicine*, Sixth Edition. Philadelphia: W. B. Saunders, 1984, 249. M. A. Conant *et al.*, "Secondary Syphilis Misdiagnosed as Infectious Mononucleosis." *California Medicine* 109:6 (1968) 462–464. D. R. Turner *et al.*, "Lymphadenopathy in Early Syphilis." *J. Pathology* 110 (1973), 305–308.

3. J. J. McKenna *et al.*, *op. cit.* USDHEW PHS, *Syphilis: Modern Diagnosis and Management*. Washington, D.C.: GPO, 1961, 28. L. M. Drusin, "The Diagnosis and Treatment of Infectious and Latent Syphilis." *Medical Clinics of North America* 56:5 (1972), 1161–1174.

4. Harold W. Jaffe, "Treatment of Latent Syphilis." *J. American Venereal Disease Association* 3:2, part 2, (1976), 143–145. E. G. Clark and N. Danbolt, *op. cit.* P. Frederick Sparling, *op. cit.* J. T. Crissey and D. A. Denenholtz, "Syphilis," *Clinics in Dermatology* 2:1 (1984), 21, 35, 59, 92, 93, 100.

5. L. M. Drusin, "Syphilis: Clinical Manifestations, Diagnosis, and Treatment."

6. USDHEW PHS, *op. cit.*, 47.

7. L. M. Drusin, "Syphilis: Clinical Manifestations, Diagnosis, and Treatment."

8. *Loc. cit.* USDHEW PHS, *op. cit.*, 32ff.

9. L. M. Drusin, "Syphilis: Clinical Manifestations, Diagnosis, and Treatment."

10. USDHEW PHS, *op. cit.*, 32ff. J. J. McKenna *et al.*, "Unmasking AIDS: Chemical Immunosuppression and Seronegative Syphilis" (unpublished). W. F. Danehower, "Penicillin Fallout and Infectious Syphilis." *Medical Clinics of North America* 48 (1964), 747–753.

11. Editorial: "Masking or Unveiling Syphilis?" *New England Journal of Medicine* 244:25 (1951), 955–956.

12. H. A. Christian, *The Principles and Practice of Medicine.* Sixteenth Edition. New York and London: D. Appleton-Century Co., 1947, 425.

13. Rene J. Dubos, ed., *Bacterial and Mycotic Infections of Man.* Third Edition. Philadelphia: Lippincott, 1958, 532.

14. W. F. Danehower, *op. cit.* D. H. Hollander *et al.*, "The Effect of Long-Continued Subcurative Doses of Penicillin During the Incubation Period of Experimental Syphilis." *Bulletin of the Johns Hopkins Hospital* 90 (1952), 105–120.

15. USDHEW PHS, *op. cit.*, 47. W. F. Danehower, *op. cit.*

16. P. Collart, *et al.*, "Modified Method of Filtering Cerebrospinal Fluid and Aqueous Humor for the Detection of Treponemes: Proof of the Persistence of Their Vitality in Rabbits." *British J. Venereal Diseases* 50 (1974), 251–256.

17. H. W. Jaffe, "Treatment of Latent Syphilis."

18. V. Lauderdale and J. N. Goldman, "Serial Ultrathin Sectioning Demonstrating the Intracellularity of *T. pallidum.*"

Brit. J. of Venereal Diseases 48 (1972), 87–96. C. N. Sowmini, "Clinical Progression of Ocular Syphilis and Neurosyphilis Despite Treatment with Massive Doses of Penicillin. Failure to Demonstrate Treponemes in Affected Tissues." *Brit. J. Venereal Diseases* 47 (1971), 348–355. J. Lawton Smith, "Spirochetes in Late Seronegative Syphilis Despite Penicillin Therapy." *Medical Times* 96 (1968), 611–623. J. D. Bos, *Immunological Aspects of Syphilis (Academisch Proefschrift)*. Amsterdam: Rodopi, 1981, 12.

19. Lawrence Altman, "AIDS May Spread Outside Bloodstream." *New York Times*, December 13, 1986, 10.

20. Editorial: "Treatment of Primary and Secondary Syphilis: Defining Failure at Three- and Six-Month Follow-up."

21. G. T. Strickland, *op. cit.*, 252. D. M. Markovitz *et al.*, "Failure of Recommended Treatment for Secondary Syphilis," *JAMA* 255:13 (1986), 1767–1768. N. J. Fiumara, "Failure of Recommended Treatment for Secondary Syphilis" (letter), *JAMA* 256:11 (1986), 1443–1444.

22. P. F. Sparling, *op. cit.* Harold W. Jaffe, "Treatment of Latent Syphilis." J. Joergensen *et al.*, "Neurosyphilis After Treatment of Latent Syphilis with Benzathine Penicillin." *Genitourin. Med.* 62 (1986), 129–131. D.J.M. Wright and J. L. Turk, "Cell-Mediated Immunity and Lymphocyte Transformation in Syphilis." *Proc. Royal Soc. Med.* 64 (1971), 426–448.

23. J. Joergensen *et al.*, *op. cit.*

24. J. L. Smith, *op. cit.* J. L. Smith and C. W. Israel, *op. cit.* L. Yogeswari and C. W. Chacko, "Persistence of *T. pallidum* and its Significance in Penicillin-Treated Seropositive Late Syphilis." *Brit. J. Venereal Diseases* 47 (1971), 339–347. A. R. Yobs *et al.*, "Treponemal Survival in Humans After Penicillin Therapy." *Brit. J. Venereal Dis-*

eases 40 (1964), 248–253. P. F. Sparling, *op. cit.* N.S.C. Rice *et al.*, "Demonstration of Treponeme-Like Forms in Cases of Treated and Untreated Late Syphilis and of treated Early Syphilis." *Brit. J. Venereal Diseases* 46 (1970), 1–9.

25. P. Collart and M. Poitevin, *op. cit.*

26. P. F. Sparling, *op. cit.*

27. W. F. Danehower, "Penicillin Fallout and Infectious Syphilis."

28. Editorial: "Treatment of Primary and Secondary Syphilis: Defining Failure at Three- and Six-Month Follow-up."

29. K. Weisman *et al.*, *op. cit.*

30. Iago Galdston, *The Impact of Antibiotics on Medicine and Society.* New York: International Universities Press, 1958, 211.

31. M. A. Conant *et al.*, "Secondary Syphilis Masquerading as Infectious Mononucleosis."

32. Armand J. Pereyra *et al.*, "A Graphic Guide for Clinical Management of Latent Syphilis," *California Medicine* 112:5 (1970), 13–18.

33. P. Collart and M. Poitevin, *op. cit.*

34. L. M. Drusin *et al.*, "Infectious Syphilis Mimicking Neoplastic Disease." *Archives of Internal Medicine* 137:2 (1977), 156–160. A. J. Pereyra *et al.*, *op. cit.* P. F. Sparling, *op. cit.*

35. Michael Specter, "Fear of AIDS Cited as Syphilis Rate Declines." *Washington Post*, August 10, 1985, A-1.

36. USDHEW PHS, *op. cit.*, 2.

37. P. F. Sparling, *op. cit.*

38. L. M. Drusin, "Syphilis: Clinical Manifestations, Diagnosis and Treatment." J. T. Crissey and D. A. Denenholtz, *op. cit.* N. J. Fiumara, *op. cit.* J. Joergensen *et al.*, *op. cit.* D. M. Markovits *et al.*, *op. cit.*

39. "Case Records of the Massachusetts General Hospital: Case 27–1983."

40. S. J. McPhee, "Secondary Syphilis: Uncommon Manifestations of a Common Disease." *Western J. Medicine* 140:1 (1984), 35. R. A. Smego *et al.*, *op. cit.* M. A. Conant *et al.*, *op. cit.* "Case Records of the Massachusetts General Hospital: Case 27:1983," *New England Journal of Medicine* 309:1 (1983), 41–43. J. J. Potterat *et al.*, *op. cit.* L. M. Drusin, "Syphilis: Clinical Manifestations, Diagnosis and Treatment." P. D. Walker *et al.*, "Rapidly Progressive Glomerulonephritis in a Patient With Syphilis." *A. J. Medicine* 76 (June, 1984), 1106–1112. E. W. Baum *et al.*, "Secondary Syphilis: Still the Great Imitator." *JAMA* 249:22 (1983), 3069–3070

41. T. A. Chapel, "Physician Recognition of the Signs and Symptoms of Secondary Syphilis." *JAMA* 246:3 (1981), 250–251.

42. J. Sonnabend *et al.*, "Acquired Immunodeficiency Syndrome, Opportunistic Infectious, and Malignancies in Male Homosexuals." *JAMA* 249:17 (1983), 2370–2374.

43. Carol Dawn Berry, M.D. *et al.*, "Neurologic Relapse After Benzathine Penicillin Therapy for Secondary Syphilis in a Patient with HIV Infection." *New England Journal of Medicine* 316:25 (1987), 1587–1589.

44. Donald R. Johns, M.D. *et al.*, "Alteration in the Natural History of Neurosyphilis by Concurrent Infection with the Human Immunodeficiency Virus." *New England Journal of Medicine* 316:25 (1987), 1569–1572.

Chapter IV — Syphilis and the Immune System

1. J. T. Crissey and D. A. Denenholz, *op. cit.*

2. Loyd Thompson, *op. cit.*, 457. J. D. Bos, *op. cit.* Jean Oliver, "Syphilitic Disease of the Thymus in Infants and the Mode of Origin of the Dubois Abscesses." A. J. *Diseases of Children* 13 (1917), 158–166. H. A. Christian, *The Principles and Practice of Medicine*, 457.

3. J. D. Bos, *op. cit.* J. T. Crissey and D. A. Denenholz, *op. cit.*

4. J. T. Crissey and D. A. Denenholz, *op. cit.*

5. J. D. Bos *et al.*, "Antitreponemal IgE in Early Syphilis." *British Journal of Venereal Diseases* 56 (1980), 20–25. J. J. Thompson *et al.*, "Immunoregulatory Properties of Serum from Patients with Different Stages of Syphilis." *British Journal of Venereal Diseases* 56 (1980), 210–217. J. R. Jensen *et al.* "Depression of Natural Killer Cell Activity by Syphilis Serum and Immune Complexes." *British Journal of Venereal Diseases* 58 (1982), 298–301.

6. Joan McKenna, *et al.*, *op. cit.* J. J. Thompson *et al.*, "Immunoregulatory Properties of Serum from Patients with Different Stages of Syphilis." *Brit. J. Venereal Diseases* 56 (1980), 210–217. D.J.M. Wright and J. L. Turk, *op. cit.* N. Clumeck *et al.*, "Heterosexual promiscuity Among African Patients with AIDS" (letter). *New England Journal of Medicine* 313:3 (1985), 182. E. From *et al.*, "Reactivity of Lymphocytes from Patients with Syphilis Towards *T. pallidum* Antigen in the Leucocyte Migration and Lymphocyte Transformation Tests." *Brit. J. Venereal Diseases* 52 (1976), 224–229.

7. J. Cohen, *op. cit.*, 254.

8. D. I. Abrams *et al.*, "Lymphadenopathy: Endpoint or Prodrome? Update of a 24-Month Prospective Study." *An-*

nals of the New York Academy of Sciences 437 (1984), 207–215.

9. *Ibid.*, 209.

10. *Ibid.*, 208.

11. *Ibid.*, 210–211.

12. J. A. Sonnabend *et al.*, "A Multifactorial Model for the Development of AIDS in Homosexual Men." Robert Elie *et al.*, "Thymic Dysplasia in Acquired Immunodeficiency Syndrome" (letter). *New England Journal of Medicine* 308:14 (1983) 841.

13. Claudia Wallis, "AIDS: A Growing Threat."

14. N. Dozier *et al.*, *op. cit.* K. Weismann *et al.*, *op. cit.*

15. J. I. Wallace *et al.*, "T-Cell Ratios in Homosexuals" (letter). *The Lancet* (April 17, 1982), 908. H. Kornfeld *et al.*, "T-Lymphocyte Subpopulations in Homosexual Men." *New England Journal of Medicine* 307:12 (1982), 729–731.

16. J. J. Goedert, *et al.*, "Amyl Nitrite May Alter T-Lymphocytes in Homosexual Men." *The Lancet* (February 29, 1982), 412–415.

17. R. Lindskov *et al.*, "Acute HTLV-III Infection with Roseola-Like Rash" (letter). *The Lancet* (February 22, 1986), 447.

18. J. J. McKenna *et al.*, *op. cit.*

19. Cristine Russell, "AIDS Virus Linked to Brain Damage." *Wahington Post*, December 12, 1985, A-1. David D. Ho *et al.*, "Isolation of HTLV-III From Cerebrospinal Fluid and Neural Tissues of Patients with Neurologic Syndromes Related to the Acquired Immunodeficiency Syndrome." *New England Journal of Medicine* 313:24 (1985), 1493–1497.

20. E. G. Clark and N. Danbolt, *op. cit.* CDC, AIDS WEEKLY SURVEILLANCE REPORT– UNITED STATES AIDS PROGRAM. June 15, 1987. J. N. Bos, *Immunological Aspects of Syphilis.*

21. Cristine Russell, "AIDS Can Be Dormant in Body, Study Says." *Washington Post,* May 16, 1985, A-15.

22. J. Crofton and A. Douglas, *Respiratory Diseases.* Third Edition (Oxford: Blackwell, 1981). M. Wolman *et al.,* "Studies on Interstitial Giant-Cell Pneumonia." *A. J. Dis. Child.* 83:5 (1952), 573–588. H. Gormsen, "On Interstitial Giant Cell Pneumonia in Infants." *Acta Pediat.* 39 (1950), 291–314. G. R. Russell *et al.,* "Primary Atypical Pneumonia in Childhood." *S. Med. J.* 45:10 (1952), 906–914. J. Nowak, "Late Pulmonary Changes in the Course of Infection with *Pneumocystis carinii.*" *Acta Med. Pol.* 7:1 (1966), 23–41.

23. P. F. Sparling, *op. cit.* M. R. Randolph, "Primary Atypical Pneumonia in Children: A Review of Thirty-Four Cases." *Conn. State M.J.* 14 (1950), 19–27.

24. G. R. Russell *et al., op. cit.*

25. G. W. Hunter, J. C. Swartzwelder, and D. F. Clyde, *Tropical Medicine.* Philadelphia: Saunders, 1976, 404–407. F. Pavlica, "The First Observation of Congenital Pneumocystic Pneumonia in a Fully Developed Stillborn Child." *Annales Paediatrici* 198 (1962) 177–184. J. Nowak, *op. cit.*

26. D. R. Perera *et al.,* "Pneumocystis carinii Pneumonia in a Hospital for Children." *JAMA* 214:6 (1970), 1074–1078.

27. J. J. McKenna *et al., op. cit.*

28. J. Nowak, *op. cit.* P. Troen, "Explosive Outbreak of an Atypical Pneumonia." *Arch. Intern. Med.* 89 (1952), 258–269. G. Williams *et al.,* "AIDS in 1959?" (letter) *The Lancet* (November 12, 1983) 1136.

29. G. Williams *et al.,* "Cytomegalic Inclusion Disease and *Pneumocystis carinii* infection in an Adult." *The Lancet* (October 28, 1960), 951–955. M. Wolman *et al., op. cit.* H. Gormsen, *op. cit.* P. Troen, *op. cit.* A. Hartung *et al.,* "Pulmonary Syphilis." JAMA 98:23 (1932), 1969–1972. N. Dozier *et al., op. cit.*

30. A. Hartung, *op. cit.* H. Schibli *et al.,* "Tumor-like Pulmonary Lesion in Secondary Syphilis." *British J. Venereal Diseases* 57 (1981), 367–371.

31. D. L. Coleman *et al.,* "Secondary Syphilis with Pulmonary Involvement." *Western J. Med.* 138:6 (1983), 875–877.

32. F. W. Chandler *et al.,* "Pulmonary Pneumocystis in Nonhuman primates."

33. B. D. Myers *et al.,* "Kaposi's Sarcoma in Kidney Transplant Patients." *Arch. Intern. Med.* 133:2 (1974), 307–311. J. H. Siegel *et al.,* "Disseminated Visceral Kaposi's Sarcoma." JAMA 207:8 (1969), 1493–1496. Editorial: "Cancer in the Immunosuppressed Patient." *Annals of Internal Medicine* 75:2 (1971), 310–312.

34. T. C. Quinn *et al.,* "AIDS in Africa: an Epidemiologic Paradigm."

35. M. Marmor *et al.,* "Risk Factors for Kaposi's Sarcoma in Homosexual Men." *The Lancet* (May 15, 1982), 1083–1087.

36. N. Dozier *et al., op. cit.* J. J. McKenna *et al., op. cit.*

37. T. C. Quinn *et al.,* "AIDS in Africa: an Epidemiologic Paradigm."

38. *Loc. cit.* R. Colebunders *et al.,* "AIDS in Patients seen with Malaria and Cryptococcosis" (letter) *Central African J. Medicine* 31:1 (1985), 17–18.

39. T. C. Quinn *et al.*, "AIDS in Africa: an Epidemologic Paradigm."

40. *Loc. cit.*

41. *Loc. cit.*

42. J. W. Curran *et al.*, *op. cit.*

43. T. C. Quinn *et al.*, "AIDS in Africa: an Epidemologic Paradigm."

44 N. Dozier *et al.*, *op. cit.* J. Cohen, *op. cit.* J. W. Curran *et al.*, *op. cit.*

45 N. Dozier *et al.*, *op. cit.* R. E. Stahl *et al.*, *op. cit.*

Chapter V — Medicinal Suppression

1. L. M. Drusin, "Syphilis: Clinical Manifestations, Diagnosis, and Treatment."

2. Editorial: "Treatment of Primary and Secondary Syphilis: Defining Failure at Three- and Six-Month Follow-up."

3. B. A. Cunha *et al.*, "Adverse Effects of Antibiotics." *Heart and Lung* 13:5 (1984), 465–472. A. G. Gilman *et al.*, *Goodman and Gilman's The Pharmacological Basis of Therapeutics*. Sixth Edition. New York: Macmillan, 1980, 1148, 1150.

4. *Ibid.*, 1147. Jack H. Dean, *Immunotoxicology and Immuno pharmacology*. New York: Raven Press, 1985, 91–98. Christian Tauchnitz and Werner Handrick, "Unerwuenschte Arzneimittelwirkungen und Arzneimittelschaeden I: Schaedigungen durch Antibiotika und Chemotherapeutika." *Zeitschrift fuer die Gesamte Innere Medizin und Ihre Grenzgebiete* 38:24 (1983) 653–659.

5. A. G. Gilman *et al.*, *op. cit.*, 1148–1149.

6. Jack H. Dean, ed., *op. cit.*, 91–98.

7. L. M. Drusin, "Syphilis: Clinical Manifestations, Diagnosis, and Treatment."

8. A. G. Gilman, *et al.*, *op. cit.*, 1188. R. Finch, "Immunomodulating Effects of Antimicrobial Agents." *J. Antimicrobial Chemotherapy* 6 (1980), 691–699.

9. A. G. Gilman *et al.*, *op. cit.*, 1188.

10. *Ibid.* 1224. R. Finch, *op. cit.*

11. J. McKenna *et al.*, *op. cit.*

12. R. Finch, *op. cit.*

13. A. G. Gilman *et al.*, *op. cit.*, 1113.

14. *Physician's Desk Reference.* Thirty-Ninth Edition (1985), 2005–2006.

15. John L. Giunta *et al.*, "Ampicillin Allergy Presenting as Secondary Syphilis." *Oral Surgery* 57:2 (1984), 152–154.

16. In D. P. Stites *et al.*, *Basic and Clinical Immunology.* Fifth Edition. Los Altos, California: Lange, 1984, 13.

17. N. Dozier *et al.*, *op. cit.* J. Cohen, *op. cit. Physician's Desk Reference.* Thirty-Ninth Edition (1985), 824, 1577, 2103.

18. J. Sonnabend *et al.*, "Acquired Immune Deficiency Syndrome, Opportunistic Infection, and Malignancies in Male Homosexuals."

19. D. J. Morton and S. A. Langton, "Antibiotic Prescribing in Zimbabwe." *Central African Journal of Medicine* 31:12 (1985), 249–250.

20. S. F. Dealler and P. R. Mason, "Sensitivity to Antibiotics of Bacteria Isolated in the Public Health Laboratory, Harare." *Central African Journal of Medicine* 31:6 (1985), 111–113.

21. T. C. Quinn *et al., op. cit.*

22. J. W. Curran *et al.,op. cit.*

23. Lawrence K. Altman, "Linking AIDS to Africa Provokes Bitter Debate."

Chapter VI—The AIDS Virus a Co-Factor?

1. Peter H. Duesberg, *op. cit.*

2. "Needlestick Transmission of HTLV-III From a Patient Infected in Africa." *The Lancet* (December 15, 1984), 1376–1377.

3. C. Neisson-Vernant *et al.,* "Needlestick HIV Seroconversion in a Nurse" (letter). *The Lancet* (October 4, 1986), 814.

4. Philip J. Hilts, "The Advocate for AIDS Testing." *Washington Post*, December 27, 1986, C-1.

5. M. S. Hirsch *et al.,* "Risk of Nosocomial Infection with Human T-Cell Lymphotropic Virus III (HTVL-III)." *New England Journal of Medicine* 312:1 (1985), 1–4.

6. M. S. Hirsh *et al.,* "Risk of Transmission of HTLV-III by Needle Stick" (letter). *New England Journal of Medicine* 312: 17 (1985), 1128–1129.

7. Personal communication from Ruth Ann Marcus of the Centers for Disease Control, Atlanta.

8. R. J. Biggar *et al.,* "Seroepidemiology of HTLV-III Antibodies in a Remote Population of Eastern Zaire." *British Medical Journal* 290 (March 16, 1985), 808–810.

9. Peter H. Duesberg, *op. cit.*

10. Lawrence K. Altman, "Third AIDS Virus Found in Sweden." *New York Times*, November 20, 1986, A-24. Michael Specter, "Discovery Indicates Link of AIDS, Monkey Virus." *Washington Post*, April 9, 1987, A-20.

11. Jane Teas, "Could AIDS Agent Be a New Variant of African Swine Fever Virus?" (letter). *The Lancet* (April 23, 1983), 923.

12. J. Beldekas *et al.*, "African Swine Fever Virus and AIDS" (letter). *The Lancet* (March 8, 1986), 564–565. Neil Miller, "The Other Theory on AIDS." *The Boston Phoenix*, June 3, 1986.

13. Lawrence K. Altman, "Studies Fail to Link AIDS with Swine Fever." *New York Times*, September 19, 1985, B-15. New York State Department of Health. Wadsworth Center for Laboratories and Research. Memorandum (unpublished) from Dr. Dickerman to Dr. Lawrence. Date: September 17, 1985. Subject: HTLV-3 and African Swine Fever (ASF).

14. Neil Miller, "The Other Theory on AIDS."

15. Kieth Schneider, "U.S. To Test for a Link of AIDS to Swine Fever." *New York Times*, July 17, 1986, 12.

16. P. Feorino *et al.*, "AIDS and African Swine Fever Virus" (letter). *The Lancet* (October 4, 1986), 815.

17. C. V. Martins *et al.*, "African Swine Fever and AIDS" (letter). *The Lancet* (June 28, 1986), 1504–1505.

18. W. A. Blattner *et al.*, "Epidemiology of Human T-Lymphotropic Virus Type III and the Risk of Acquired Immunodeficiency Syndrome." *Annals of Internal Medicine* 103 (1985), 665–670.

19. J. L. Levy and J. L. Ziegler, "Acquired Immunodeficiency Syndrome is an Opportunistic Infection, and Kaposi's Sarcoma Results from Secondary Immune Stimulation." *The Lancet* (July 9, 1983), 79–81.

20. Peter H. Duesberg, *op. cit.*

21. Quoted in Jonathan Lieberson, "The Reality of AIDS." *New York Review of Books* (January 16, 1986), 43–48.

22 *Loc. cit.*

Chapter VII—Prevention and Treatment

1. Editorial: "The Weiss Watch." *Wall Street Journal,* April 29, 1987, 30.

2. H. C. Lane *et al.,* "Immunologic Reconstitution in the Acquired Immunodeficiency Syndrome." *Annals of Internal Medicine* 102 (1985), 714–718.

3. Laurence Badgley, M.D., "Homeopathy for Acquired Immune Deficiency Syndrome (A.I.D.S.)." *Journal of the American Institute of Homeopathy* 80:1 (1987), 8–14. On homoeopathy generally, see H. L. Coulter, *Homoeopathic Medicine.* St. Louis: Formur, 1972; H. L. Coulter, *Homoeopathic Science and Modern Medicine.* Berkeley, California: North Atlantic Press, 1981; George Vithoulkas, *The Science of Homeopathy, a Modern Textbook.* New York: Grove Press, 1979. H. L. Coulter, *Divided Legacy: The Conflict Between Homoeopathy and the American Medical Association.* Richmond, California: North Atlantic Books, 1982.

4. Personal communication from Guru Sandesh Singh Khalsa, N.D., Staff Supervisor of the ARC and AIDS Clinic of the National College of Naturopathic Medicine, Portland, Oregon.

5. Personal communication from Maurice Jenaer, M.D.

6. Personal communication from Guru Sandesh Singh Khalsa, N.D.

7. Laurence Badgley, M.D., *Healing AIDS Naturally: Natural Therapies for the Immune System.* San Bruno, California: Human Energy Press, 1986.

8. Robert E. Pollack, "For a National Effort to Develop a Vaccine to Counteract AIDS." *New York Times,* November 27, 1985, Op-Ed page. "Group Tells of a Step Toward AIDS Vaccine." *New York Times,* December 5, 1986, A-19.